THE
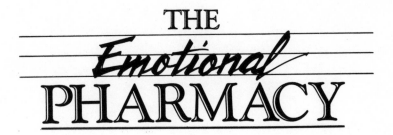
Emotional
PHARMACY

by

Roberta Morgan

THE BODY PRESS

To the spirit that can bring peace of mind

©1988 Roberta Morgan

Published by The Body Press
A division of Price Stern Sloan, Inc.
360 N. La Cienega Blvd.
Los Angeles, CA 90048

First Printing
Manufactured in the United States of America

Library of Congress Cataloging-in-Publication data

Morgan, Roberta A.
  The emotional pharmacy.

  Bibliography: p.
  Includes index.
  1. Psychotropic drugs. 2. Drug abuse. 3. Mental
illness—Chemotherapy. I. Title.
RM315.M67   1988   615'.788   88-2875
ISBN 0-89586-709-5
ISBN 0-89586-708-7 (pbk.)

ACKNOWLEDGMENTS

I would like to thank the following people and organizations for their special assistance in the research, preparation, and editing of this book:

Samuel Mitnick and Judith Wesley Allen of The Body Press; Agnes Birnbaum of Bleecker Street Associates; Dr. Bernard Salzman; Rev. Gene Orteneau; Jim Heagy, Senior Forensic Chemist, the Drug Enforcement Administration (DEA); Darrell S. Miles, Phoenix House Foundation, Inc.; the DEA; Narcotic and Drug Research, Inc.; D.I.N. Publications; Marianne Estes, Drug Program Analyst, State of California, Department of Drug and Alcohol Programs; and the American Council for Drug Education (ACDE).

Finally, I would like to especially thank my husband, Dr. Brian L.G. Morgan of Columbia University, for his invaluable help with assembling Part Two of this book, as well as for his never-ending, never-failing love, support and inspiration.

LIST OF ILLUSTRATIONS

CONTRIBUTING ARTISTS

Pages 17, 18 and 121: Illustrations by Lauren Keswick and art direction and conceptualization by John W. Karapelou of Audio-Visual Service, College of Physicians and Surgeons, Columbia University, New York.

Page 122: Illustrations, art direction, and conceptualization by John W. Karapelou.

Pages 199 and 201: Illustrations by Angela La Valle.

CONTENTS

Preface

The information you are about to read is in no way meant to be a substitute for professional diagnosis and treatment. Should you feel that you suffer from one of the emotional disorders discussed, or if you are already under the care of a physician and wish to change your method of treatment in some way, consult a qualified psychiatrist or psychologist. Similarly, if the abuse of psychoactive drugs has affected your behavior and health, you should find an experienced and state-licensed treatment program, or consult a doctor well-versed in such matters.

Having said that, I would now like to stress what I see as the importance of this book. First of all, there are currently precious few volumes that deal with psychological problems and treatment in a way that is understandable and useful for the layman. Many people talk about mental disorders, may joke about their "neuroses," and consider therapy to be a natural fixture of modern life. Yet at the same time few people truly understand the concepts and techniques used in analysis, principally the remarkable breakthroughs made in the last decade through the use of psychoactive medications.

Furthermore, an increasing number of people are being placed on these drugs to treat emotional problems—a general practitioner may even be the first one to prescribe them—and yet many of these patients are unsure of what they are taking, why drugs have been prescribed, and what the possible side effects might be. They may not be familiar with drug-nutrient interactions (how the medication can affect your nutritional status) or drug-drug interactions (how taking one drug with another can change the overall effect, or actually be dangerous).

The new age of mental chemistry has changed the nature of psychiatric treatment. In many cases, what was once a long and costly procedure has been shortened to one that is considerably less involved and expensive. People who might have been hospitalized in the past are now able to function in the outside world. Major and minor symptoms of mental illness may be effectively alleviated through the use of psychoactive drugs while therapy is going on.

However, all great breakthroughs in history have invoked controversy. Critics of chemical treatment say that patients may become dependent on psychoactive drugs and never get to the root of their problems; they also say that seriously ill patients may be given medication and sent out of hospitals into the street, where many become part of the homeless population. Both the pros and cons of chemical treatment will be examined in this book.

The most significant "con" in any type of psychoactive drug use is its potential for abuse. Both illicit drugs and prescription drugs, if used improperly or excessively, have the ability to cause as much illness as prescribed medicines can cure. This is another vital issue affecting society today which everyone should understand, and no book about drugs that affect the mind would be complete without an examination of drugs of abuse.

In order to cover these topics, this book has been divided into three parts. The first discusses the history that led us into this new age of drug treatment, the reasons why drug therapy works, and the causes and symptoms of various types of emotional illnesses that are treated with drugs. The second part examines the approximately 50 different generic types of medication (brand names in each entry are listed with the generic title) used in treatment. This section provides history, uses, side effects, dosage levels, and other relevant information about each drug. Part Three deals with drugs of abuse, explaining how each is used, why it is used, its mental and physical side effects, the possibility of long-term damage, and options for treatment.

To present an unbiased overview of the use of psychoactive drugs, the information in this book has been compiled from extensive research and numerous interviews with psychiatrists and psychologists. This information is an overview—a summary—and not an in-depth explanation of the field of psychiatry, which would fill many volumes larger than this one.

Psychology is a growing and creative field, and there are many differing opinions as to diagnosis and care. Because each person is an individual with specific problems, no form of treatment can arbitrarily be deemed the right one for every situation. This book tries to present a combination of many views and possible treatments; there may be others that are just as valid.

At one time or another in our lives, many of us may encounter problems—most of them minor—that affect our emotional health. I hope this book will serve as a guide that takes the fear and confusion out of the process of seeking help, and reassures people that immediate and effective relief is more easily found than ever before.

R.M.
New York City

PART ONE

THE ILLNESSES

INTRODUCTION:
A New Age

Almost two decades ago, I was a resident counselor in my college dormitory. This meant I was responsible for the general health and well-being of about ten women who lived on my floor. One night, I was awakened by one of them. She frantically explained that her roommate had not left the room for several weeks, complaining of severe anxiety, and now said she felt as though she was having a heart attack. We rushed this girl to the hospital, where I was eventually told that the problem was a psychiatric one—she was suffering from severe anxiety attacks (now commonly called panic attacks) and agoraphobia, which prevented her from leaving familiar surroundings.

I observed the girl for a period of almost a year, during which time she underwent extensive psychotherapy, seeing her analyst as many as four times a week. She continued to have severe attacks and found it hard to go out of doors. Although these symptoms eventually subsided with time and treatment, that year for her was time in hell.

About a year ago, before beginning this book, I encountered the same situation again. Ryan is a writer and a close personal friend. Without warning he began to suffer from severe panic attacks and agoraphobia. He couldn't write, couldn't sleep for more than a few hours at a time, and lost his appetite. We both feared he would have to endure a long, painful and expensive period of recovery. But we were very wrong. During Ryan's first visit with his therapist, they discussed the problems he was currently facing that might have caused his attacks, and he was given a prescription for a drug called Xanax (alprazolam), an antianxiety agent with mild antidepressant action that can relieve panic attacks. Finances were discussed, and the psychiatrist agreed to see Ryan once every two weeks. Due to the Xanax, Ryan's panic attacks disappeared while this therapy was ongoing, and in less than a year he was able to discontinue both medication and therapy. Today, Ryan is a successful novelist who suffers from none of his previous anxiety.

The difference between these two cases clearly illustrates the advantages of the new forms of psychiatric treatment and the introduction of chemical therapy. Ryan did not have to suffer during the interim period before the problem was solved. He could write and get on with his life. The amount of time he needed to spend with his therapist was also decreased, causing less financial hardship.

But these new advances have even more far-reaching significance. Psychiatry was once considered something less than a science because it was thought to have no biological or chemical basis. Its illnesses appeared to stem from arbitrary theories of behavior rather than organic problems. Then along came brain research, and all that changed. Scientists found that the brain, like other organs of the body, was subject to imbalances, and some forms of mental illness were no different from physical illness. Previously, many people thought the mentally ill "talked themselves into it" or were inherently "weak." Today we find that upsets in the chemical balance of the neurotransmitters (chemical messengers) in the brain, some of these even genetically transmitted, may be the cause of emotional disorders. With the knowledge that chemicals are at work, the logical conclusion is that chemicals—in the form of various medications—can be used to correct the symptoms.

When the symptoms of disorders are relieved, it is often easier for the patient to face his problems and improve more quickly. Also, people with serious disorders were once locked in institutions and the figurative keys were thrown away. No more. With medication, many people can leave the hospital and begin to lead normal lives.

Many experts believe that through these new methods more people can be treated and cured. The sometimes prohibitive costs of therapy have been reduced to a more affordable level. And what seemed to be a long, dark road toward health—therapy that could last a decade—has changed in many cases to a short-term, immediate treatment of pressing problems. Through the use of drugs such as lithium carbonate, for example, manic-depressives (now called bipolar patients) need not suffer from crippling mood swings that disrupt their lives. People unable to work or communicate with others because of severe depression can regain their interest in life through the use of antidepressant medications.

However, psychoactive drugs are a mixed blessing. Some doctors are wary of this new age of chemical therapy, although they may use some drugs to relieve certain problems. Their complaints may be valid. They say many of these drugs don't *cure* anything, they just eliminate the symptoms, so those who take them without simultaneously undergoing therapy may never solve their root problems. These people can become "pharmacopaths," they warn, needing medication for the rest of their lives. Others believe that people can develop a psychological dependence on the drugs, believing they will never get better if their medications are taken away.

Some complaints are even more serious. Many people blame these drugs for the growing number of homeless individuals, some of whom are patients released from institutions because medication has made them so "docile" that hospitalization seems unnecessary. However, they are not competent enough to hold jobs or find places to live. A few critics have accused society of becoming as it was in the Middle Ages, when the insane were sent out to wander through the wilderness and eventually die.*

Another serious complaint is that many of these medications must be taken at specific times of the day, both for effectiveness and safety. People who are seriously ill can forget or refuse to take their medications without supervision, causing their disturbed behavior to return and possibly becoming threats to themselves or others. Some patients play "catch up"—they take three pills at once because they have forgotten to take the others at their proper times. With certain drugs, this can cause toxic reactions.

Some psychiatrists complain that clinics may dispense medication without requiring follow-up therapy. They also say that psychoactive medications are sometimes prescribed by doctors not skilled in psychiatry, leading to treatment with the wrong type or strength of drug, again without accompanying therapy.

Finally, some of these drugs are very powerful, and can have disturbing side effects and sedative effects. There is a group of people who believe that the stronger drugs, such as certain antipsychotics, should only be used as a last resort.

One cannot deny that the critics make some valid points, but the benefits of using these drugs in most cases appear to outweigh the dangers. As a compromise measure to solve some of the problems, perhaps seriously ill patients should remain hospitalized and doctors in all specialties should insist that adequate therapy always accompany the use of psychoactive drugs.

The important thing to remember is that the whole field of psychiatry has changed, and people can be helped more easily than ever before. Granted, we are still unsure of the exact causes of mental illness, and the number of people who can be "cured"—especially the seriously ill—is still not impressive. However, the combination of new forms of therapy

* New laws designed to safeguard patients' rights have sometimes added to this problem. The Lanterman-Petris-Short Act of 1967 determined that a person could be detained in a residential psychiatric treatment program only if he was a danger to himself or others. Hence, the number of mental patients in U.S. institutions shrank from a peak of about 560,000 in 1955 to approximately 146,000 in 1984.

and research in the field of brain chemistry is helping to uncover clues that may one day—perhaps in the near future—make mental illness a thing of the past.

CHAPTER ONE

FINDING THE KEYS:
A Brief History of Psychiatric and Chemical Treatment

As we all know, our ancestors were not kind to the victims of mental illness. Although depression and other emotional problems were described in the Old Testament and by both the Romans and Greeks, people had little understanding of, or sympathy for, such disorders. They were attributed to strange causes (a wandering uterus, angry gods), and the sufferers were often cast out of the community, left to wander without help and die alone.

The picture grew even darker before it improved. Many mentally ill people were accused of being possessed by demons in medieval times. They were tortured, burned at the stake, or paraded around to invoke horror and/or amusement from spectators. This entertainment factor continued in later centuries, when the curious could pay admission to mental institutions, and laugh and taunt the ill-treated patients who were behind bars or chained to the walls. Some villages chose to drive them into the hills, where only the most competent could survive.

In the La Bicêtre Hospital in Paris, during the 18th century, horrible sights would await a visitor's eyes. Chronically insane patients were normally shackled to the walls of dark cells, held fast by iron collars or iron hoops around the waist, arms, and legs. Many of them could not even lie down at night. The food they were served was often spoiled; their cells contained little but straw and were never cleaned out. No one visited the cells except at feeding time, and then attendants did not show even a glimmer of warmth or consideration for the patients.

History also shows us that the use of drugs to alter mental states is nothing new, although in ancient times, drugs were used primarily for religious rites. The Incas were very fond of the coca plant (the natural form of cocaine), and other populations frequently used opiates, herb derivatives, and similar concoctions as an integral part of their lives. In fact, the derivatives of a plant called rauwolfia had been used for centuries in India to treat many illnesses—including mental illness. It took the West until 1931 to find that rauwolfia serpentina could be used to help psychiatric patients.

A few major revolutions in psychiatric history paved the way for our current attitudes and treatment of the mentally ill. The first was in the late 18th century, when Phillippe Pinel and others established mental asylums and used them to house and treat the insane. They humanized the way people were handled in these institutions and recognized that the mentally ill were suffering from a disease.

Probably the best known historical figure in the field of psychiatry is Sigmund Freud (1856-1939). Many of our current beliefs about behavioral development and psychopathology originated with the work of Freud, who created psychoanalytic theory and therapy. His account of unconscious mental processes has had a dramatic effect on our society and science, although many of his theories have now been discarded and his techniques modified. But few know that the young Freud would have been thrilled by the concept of treating emotional illness with drugs, because it would have validated his initial theories. Freud was a neurologist who started out believing that psychological problems were neurological in origin and had their basis in the structure and function of the brain. In 1875 he presented his study of the effects of cocaine on the mind. Although he later abandoned these theories in his practice because research techniques at the time were not advanced enough to help him prove his suspicions, his original concept that emotional illness was physical illness of the brain proved to be basically correct—with one exception. We now understand that it is not the neurons, or nerve cells in the brain, that are out of balance, but the chemicals they secrete to pass messages, such as the neurotransmitters.

In later years Freud repudiated his early ideas and came to believe that the analytic process was the only means to a cure. He divided the personality and drives into several different parts, and tried to discover how and why these parts stopped working together when a person became psychologically ill. He also felt that the major development of the adult personality took place in infancy and early childhood.

Another significant figure in the field of psychology was Carl Jung (1871-1961), who made many contributions to our current fund of knowledge. He believed psychiatric treatment should deal with current problems and plans for the future, as well as with attempts to discover the past causes of illness.

Adolf Meyer (1866-1950), who influenced many American therapists, felt that the patient should evaluate his situation and responses to life with a therapist, and then the two of them could formulate a way of dealing with the patient's problems more constructively. He introduced the concept of "common-sense psychiatry," which meant understanding the patient in the simplest terms possible. His emphasis was on solving present problems instead of delving into past ones, and helping the patient develop better habits of behavior.

Meyer could be said to be the forerunner of behavior therapists, who see mental problems as the outcome of experiences in which incorrect learning, particularly emotional learning, has occurred. For example, a child who is loved and cared for by his parents only when he is ill could develop psychiatric symptoms of illness in later life because he feels this will bring him love and attention—even though on a conscious level he is not aware of what he is doing and why.

John B. Watson (1878-1958), an American psychologist, developed a concept known as behaviorism. He believed that psychology should be the study of observable behavior and should avoid references to un-observable mental functions such as consciousness. In 1920, Watson demonstrated through a one-year-old boy named Albert that fears could be induced by conditioning behavior. Albert became fearful of a white rat, which had not frightened him previously, when a loud noise was made behind him while he was playing with the rat. After a few trials, Albert became fearful of any white rat, even without the noise, and his fear spread to other kinds of animals and objects.

Watson's trials paved the way for the work of Mary Jones and B.F. Skinner, who found that a conditioned response such as fear could be eliminated by a reverse conditioning process. Skinner developed tech-niques for demonstrating how the consequences of an act influenced a person's tendency to repeat that act. In his concept of operant condition-ing he said that a response to an act was reinforcement, and an act that was reinforced would be repeated, and vice versa. A sample experiment allowed a subject (a rat) to perform a random act (pressing down a lever). If the act resulted in the delivery of food (a reinforcer), the subject increasingly repeated the act. If nothing happened when the act was repeated (no reinforcement), the number of times the subject committed the act decreased (extinction). In the same way, people can be con-ditioned to eliminate unproductive behavior by not receiving reinforce-ment when the behavior occurs.

From these and many other pioneers in the field, the diverse types of therapy we have today developed (see Chapter Four). Many of these early ideas were modified or built upon, some were discarded, and others are still in use. With the growth in techniques for therapeutic treatment, a new kind of therapy—psychopharmacology, or the use of drugs to erase the symptoms of mental illness—appeared.

Practitioners in the field today often use a combination of different therapies and tailor their treatment to the needs of individual patients.

The Chemical Revolution

If Pinel changed the face of psychiatry in one way, and Freud in another, the use of psychoactive drugs similarly altered everything. Now psychiatric illness could be looked at as having some biochemical basis, which opened the possibility for chemical treatment. In the case of disorders such as manic-depression, drugs have managed to prevent recurrences to an extent rarely achieved before by any other type of therapy. With other disorders, medication has been shown to relieve symptoms to such a degree that the therapeutic process is enhanced in many ways, bringing about more rapid cure. If a person with an anxiety disorder can be calmed through the use of drugs, he can often communicate his problems more effectively to the therapist.

People were experimenting with drugs to affect the mind in the late 19th century, but in 1931, the reports that treatment with rauwolfia serpentina helped mental problems ushered in a new age. While it may have taken almost 40 years to fully develop, the first inroads had been made.

In the 1930s, procedures such as insulin shock and electroconvulsive therapy became available to treat major depression and schizophrenia. (The latter term refers to a group of disorders—usually psychotic in proportion—marked by certain disturbances in language, communication, thought, perception, mood and behavior that could lead to a misinterpretation of reality, and sometimes delusions and hallucinations.) Although these techniques of treatment endured, drug therapy is now often used in their place.

The research confirming a chemical basis for illness and treatment was furthered in 1943 by Dr. Albert Hofmann, a chemist working at Sandoz laboratories (a pharmaceutical firm in Basel, Switzerland). Dr. Hofmann was doing research using derivatives of the drug ergot, and one morning manufactured a few milligrams of a substance known as d-lysergic acid diethylamide, or LSD-25. He developed strange psychological symptoms, such as visions of color and feelings of mild dizziness, while working with the substance. One day he ingested what he thought was a small amount of LSD to see if the drug was causing these symptoms. For the next few hours, Hofmann embarked on one of the first well-recorded instances of an "acid trip," experiencing sensory distortions and full-blown hallucinations. While he recovered from his symptoms, his findings did demonstrate that a toxic chemical could significantly affect the functioning of the mind. Not long afterward, in 1949, an Australian doctor named John F. Cade reported that the chemical lithium could effectively treat psychotic excitement, or mania.

The first antipsychotic drug, chlorpromazine (Thorazine) was made in France in 1950, and by 1952 doctors were testing its effects on psychiatric patients. During the same period, the term "tranquilizer" was coined by a Dr. Yonkman to describe the effects of a drug called reserpine (a derivative of rauwolfia).

The field of psychopharmacology now expanded rapidly. The year 1954 saw reports on a drug called meprobamate, which marked the beginning of the invention of modern sedatives with useful antianxiety effects. Also in the 1950s, an antitubercular drug called iproniazid was discovered and found to have antidepressant effects, by stopping the action of an enzyme called monoamine oxidase. This eventually led to the use of a class of drugs now known as monoamine oxidase inhibitors (MAOIs) to treat depression. In 1958, another major class of antidepressants, the tricyclics (TCAs), was introduced with the discovery of the effects of a drug called imipramine.

Anxiety and insomnia were first treated with barbiturates, which proved too strong, too dangerous, and too likely to become habit-forming. But in 1957, a drug called chlordiazepoxide was introduced. It belonged to a chemical group called the benzodiazepines, which are now used for many anxiety-related problems. Just one year later, a new antipsychotic drug called haloperidol was discovered and led to the expansion of the types of drugs used to treat more serious mental disorders.

Throughout the 1960s, research intensified in the field of psychoactive medications. The drugs discovered in the 1950s were confirmed effective in treating patients, and new drugs were introduced.

Where We Stand Today

On the therapeutic front, much has changed since the days of Freud. In 1980, the American Psychiatric Association released the diagnostic tool, the *DSM-III (Diagnostic and Statistical Manual)* that is now used to classify and understand mental disorders. It differed from its predecessor, the *DSM-II*, in that it broke down problems into five components, or axes. It is pointless to go through them all—an example will suffice. Axis I deals with clinical syndromes, which includes all psychiatric disorders except for personality and developmental disorders— the latter are on Axis II. The second Axis can be used to uncover an underlying disorder. A patient may be diagnosed as manic-depressive on Axis I and as having a compulsive personality disorder on Axis II. Treatment can then include more than one approach in order to sort out all the problems contributing to a patient's symptoms. The revised and updated *DSM-III* was published in 1987, and is now known as the *DSM-III-R*.

Psychoactive drug treatment has brought us a long way. The year 1958 marked the first time in a century that the number of people admitted to mental hospitals (because they could no longer be treated on the outside) decreased. By 1973, admissions were down in this country to approximately 300,000, when 600,000 had been the projected figure.

Research into the chemical nature, structure, and function of the brain fully bloomed in the 1970s and 1980s, shedding much light on the psychopharmacological field. Attention focused on two of the chemicals in the brain that affect behavior—serotonin and norepinephrine. Researchers are now trying to find out to what extent disturbances in the levels of these brain chemicals are responsible for certain types of mental illness, and if drugs can be used to correct such imbalances. The scientific community is also learning more about the action of psychoactive drugs—their side effects, the risks of toxic effects, and the lengths of time they can be safely used on a patient—in order to refine their use in treatment.

There is still a long way to go, but the goal is in sight. Mental illness is less of a mystery every day, distressing symptoms can be overcome with the careful use of drugs, and other types of therapy have become quicker and more sophisticated. Someone in the near future may be able to write: "Mental illness is now easily curable."

CHAPTER TWO

The Causes of Mental Illness

Laura, a popular and intelligent 18-year-old high school student in the best of health, told her school friends she thought she was losing her mind. For a year, she had been experiencing episodes where she felt "outside herself." These sensations were accompanied by a "dead" feeling in her body. In addition, she was unsure of her balance and coordination during the attacks, and often fell into the furniture; this symptom frequently appeared when other people were around and she became slightly anxious. During these episodes, Laura did not feel in control of her body, and her thoughts were "foggy."

This mysterious illness became increasingly distressing to the young girl. Her attacks lasted from three to four hours and occurred about twice a week. Although her school grades remained stable, other parts of her life deteriorated. She had several attacks while driving a car and so stopped driving unless someone went with her. She told her boyfriend about the problem, and he began to distance himself from her and started dating other people. She finally confided in her parents and they brought her for psychiatric help.

Laura was diagnosed as having depersonalization disorder, characterized by an alteration in the perception or the experience of the self so that the usual sense of one's own reality is lost. It can be a symptom of a variety of mental disorders, such as schizophrenic, anxiety, affective, personality, and organic mental disorders. However, mild depersonalization occurs at some time in a large number of young adults, and in such cases is not diagnosed as a serious problem. When, as in Laura's case, this symptom appears in the absence of a more serious disorder, and is severe enough to disrupt a person's social or working life, the diagnosis of depersonalization disorder is made. Laura's therapist now had to address himself to the question of why the illness had affected her at that time in her life, when everything seemed to be going so smoothly.

Our knowledge about the causes of mental illness is not terribly comforting—at this point, the causes are unknown or not totally understood. What we do understand is that certain factors can play a role in the development of mental disorders. We also can examine and try to understand mental illnesses by examining symptoms of each. Research into the mechanics of the human brain yields additional clues; chemical imbalances, either from hereditary tendencies or from some external or internal forms of stress, appear to be possible culprits.

Many doctors believe that mental problems result from the interaction of the personality with either precipitating factors or predisposing factors—or usually a combination of both.

What are Precipitating Factors?

Precipitating factors are events that precede the actual start of the illness and can happen at any point in a person's life. They may range from mild upsets (an argument with a lover) to major stressors (the death of a spouse, the loss of a job), and can cause illnesses in people who are even mildly susceptible to them. For example, a schizophrenic can become hysterical after a simple disagreement with a friend, while a stable person may develop only mild anxiety after being involved in a minor car accident.

Precipitating factors include:

1. Family interactions, such as engagement, marriage, marital arguments and separations, divorce, death, pregnancy, disagreements with a child, a child's illness.

2. Social interactions, such as problems with friends, neighbors, or business associates.

3. Changes in financial status, work status or living arrangements.

4. Legal affairs, such as being sued, suing, or being arrested.

5. Occupational hazards, such as exposure to coal dust or other harmful chemicals.

6. Physical illness, infection or handicaps; starvation or malnutrition; severe physical or mental trauma; sensory deprivations; lack of sleep.

7. Drug or alcohol abuse.

What is a Predisposing Factor?

These factors make someone vulnerable or susceptible to illness and are often present throughout the person's lifetime. If these elements in the personality are severe, even minor precipitating factors can trigger an illness.

Predisposing factors include genetics, age and gender.

Genetics—Certain genes or gene combinations can make a person susceptible to specific disorders. For instance, recent research has revealed a specific genetic site that may be responsible for the appearance of manic-depressive disorders. An illness can lie dormant, however, until an outside "precipitating factor" appears. For example, some doctors feel that a tendency toward depressive illness can be inherited. Melissa, who sought help for extreme bouts of depression that began to appear after her divorce, later told her doctor that both her father and grandmother had committed suicide for no apparent reason. A well-known example of this phenomenon might be Marilyn Monroe, who suffered from mood swings and whose mother required hospitalization for mental problems.

The appearance of schizophrenic disorders is much more common in the children of schizophrenics than in the general population. However, it is still unclear whether the child's genes are responsible or whether it is the distorted environment in which the child grows up which is to blame.

Age—Certain periods of life contain special types of stress factors, not only because of the physical changes occurring at these times, but also because of the psychological problems that can come to light. Periods of special stress include adolescence, middle age, and old age.

Gender—As a rule, more women than men consult therapists, but this is not to say that more women are ill—merely that women may be less hesitant to seek help. The incidence of certain types of disorders is more common in women than men, although no illness is exclusively confined to one gender or the other. Affective (mood) disorders, such as depression, appear to be more common in women; alcoholism is more common in men. In the U.S., more suicide attempts are made by women, but more successful attempts are made by men.

Overall, the causes of mental illness should be looked at as a complex tapestry where genetic, social, and physical factors are interwoven. Some of the factors may be inborn, others may develop so early in life that they become an integral part of the personality, while others may appear relatively late in life.

Some people argue that the source of mental illness is an individual's inability to adapt to life and to his own desires. Others say that it is no more and no less than a disease of the central nervous system, and that such malfunctions are often inherited. Both views are probably too narrow, and the actual truth lies somewhere in between.

Defense Mechanisms and the Cause of Illness
We all have ways of coping with the stresses of life. Some are healthy and productive, while others can lead to symptoms of emotional illness. The conscious efforts we employ to maintain a psychological balance are called *coping mechanisms. Defense mechanisms* are outside the boundaries

of our awareness. Most of our daily frustrations and conflicts can be taken care of through the use of conscious and deliberate coping mechanisms. More complex stresses and problems may be dealt with through unconscious defense mechanisms. These unconscious defenses are not in themselves a problem, unless they are used so frequently they distort reality or limit the flexibility of our behavior. Then they may lead to abnormal psychological symptoms. Following are explanations of some specific defense mechanisms.

Repression is the *involuntary*, automatic banishment of unacceptable feelings, ideas, or impulses (such as the hatred of, or violent thoughts about, one's own parents) into the unconscious. *Displacement* is the redirection of an emotion from the original subject to a more acceptable substitute (such as the redirection of hatred toward one's parents to one's boss). *Repression plus displacement* produces phobias, or fears, which cover up the repressed wish. Carla, a 19-year-old unwed mother, became terribly afraid her two-year-old son would get very sick and die. This fear was a defense against her repressed hostility toward, and rejection of, her unconsciously unwanted child.

A *conversion disorder* is present if the primary symptom is a loss of, or change in, physical functioning that appears to be caused by a physical illness, but is instead an expression of a psychological need or conflict. *Repression plus conversion* often produces physical symptoms. Tom, a young soldier, developed paralysis of his right hand when trying to fire a gun. This was a defense against his repressed and violent hatred toward his father. If he could use the gun, he might turn it on his own parent.

Conflicts such as these, which remain repressed, do not lose their intensity simply because they have been moved into the unconscious. Because they are still so powerful, they seem to break out of the mind in other, ways—sometimes causing the symptoms of mental illness.

Other examples of the many types of defenses include *suppression*, where unacceptable feelings or behavior are *consciously* removed from a person's thoughts and feelings. The man who has consumed too much alcohol at the office Christmas party and ends up making a fool of himself may consciously try to forget what happened that night. *Regression* occurs when a person unconsciously wants to return to an earlier time in his emotional development when things were more pleasant. Barry, a happy, toilet-trained eight-year-old, temporarily lost his bladder and bowel control when his new sister arrived in the house. Gene was promoted to vice-president, but his new responsibilities made him so anxious and fearful, he began to make serious mistakes on the job and asked to be returned to his former position.

There are many other types of defenses that people use, and it is not necessary to cite all of them here. It is enough to say that these defense mechanisms, by obscuring the true problem from conscious thought, can develop into symptoms of mental disorders.

The Chemical Basis of Mental Illness: Why Drugs Help

It is necessary at this point to understand how certain areas of brain research have helped us to better understand the mechanisms behind mental illness. This information will also explain why psychoactive drugs can help in the treatment and management of emotional disorders and their accompanying symptoms.

The central nervous system (CNS)—the brain and spinal cord—can be influenced in many ways, but direct effects are caused by two types of substances, *neurotransmitters* and *neuropeptides*. Neurotransmitters are the brain's chemical messengers, released from one cell to carry (or block) information to the next cell. Neurotransmitters are secreted by neurons (nerve cells), and they carry messages to other neurons and from one area of the brain to another (see Figure 1).

FIGURE 1 Neuron

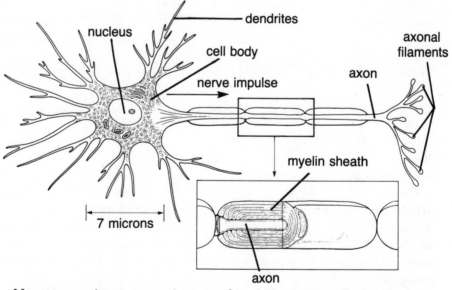

Neurotransmitters can activate or deactivate nerve cells for short or long periods of time, which can increase or decrease the number of messages being passed around the brain. This action directly influences behavior. For example, certain types of depression have been linked to a low level of catecholamines, a category of neurotransmitters. Depression may be temporarily relieved through the use of a small amount of a drug that raises the levels of catecholamines for a short period of time.

Neurotransmitter activity has a particular sequence. First, these chemicals are made and stored within the nerve cells (see Figure 2). Their release occurs when neurons are stimulated by their surroundings to the point of "firing." These chemical messengers activate the next nerve cell in the line, and are then broken down in the synaptic gap between the neurons or are reabsorbed into the neuron for later use. Some transmitters stimulate other neurons; others inhibit them. Stimulation of a neuron increases behavioral activity, inhibition slows it down or stops it.

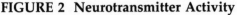

FIGURE 2   Neurotransmitter Activity

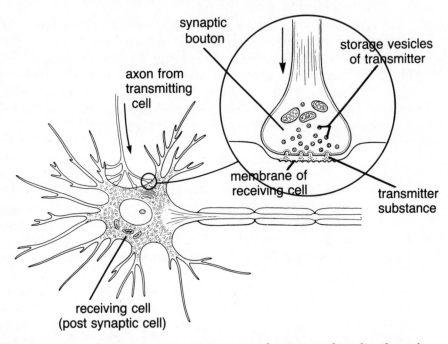

Psychoactive drugs can increase or decrease the levels of neurotransmitters in the brain. Not only is the quantity of these transmitters important to behavior, but their relative levels to each other are also significant. Several neurotransmitters have been identified as active in the CNS, and others are still being investigated. It is now believed that there may be as many as 60, 70 or more of these behavior-influencing chemicals.

The neurotransmitters about which the most is known are:

- Acetylcholine
- Norepinephrine
- Dopamine
- Serotonin
- Gamma Aminobutyric Acid (GABA)
- Glycine

The neurotransmitters called *biogenic amines* are the ones that have been implicated as playing a role in schizophrenic and affective (mood) disorders such as manic-depression. These include serotonin (in a chemical category called indoleamines), and norepinephrine and dopamine (catecholamines).

Neuropeptides, which also affect behavior, are chemicals similar to neurotransmitters. Over 20 of these are being seriously investigated, with special attention focusing on the opioid peptides (those that produce opium-like effects)—called endorphins and enkephalins. They modulate a person's response to pain and emotional distress.

All of this information has led to some sound theories as to what might be behind certain mental disorders and why particular chemicals can be used to relieve their symptoms. The biogenic amines theory of depression is one such explanation. Here, depression is assumed to reflect a reduced effective level of biogenic amines in the brain. Reserpine, a drug which was once used as an antipsychotic agent, reduces the levels of serotonin, norepinephrine and dopamine in patients. (It is no longer widely used because in many cases it caused clinical depression.) The main category of antidepressants, the tricyclics, block the re-uptake of biogenic amines from the synapses, thus elevating mood by increasing their concentration in the brain. Mood-lifters such as amphetamines and cocaine stimulate the release of catecholamines (although they do not effectively alter mood in seriously depressed patients). Pharmacological studies have suggested that some depressions may be related to a low level of norepinephrine, while others are caused by a deficiency in serotonin. Even food therapy has to some degree reinforced this theory. Many depressed people crave carbohydrates and feel better after eating them. A diet high in carbohydrates results in a boost in brain serotonin levels.

As you can see, we have only part of this chemical picture, but it is enough to suggest that the issue should be studied further. Although outside stress factors cannot be eliminated by the use of chemicals, imbalances in the brain arising out of these events, or caused by biological problems or predispositions, may one day be a thing of the past because of new drugs that manipulate abnormal levels of brain chemicals. When this is the case, it is also conceivable that the incidence and duration of mental disorders will be reduced dramatically.

CHAPTER THREE

The Symptoms of Mental Illness

Christopher, a college teacher in his mid-30s, went to his family doctor complaining of "disruptive thoughts" that kept him from studying his lecture notes or doing any kind of academic work. He said that he would constantly think about the events of the day, worrying about things he might have done wrong. He told the doctor that he would replay incidents as if they were on a videotape, asking himself if he behaved properly and telling himself that he had done his very best, or had said the right thing at all times. Sometimes hours would pass in this fashion. He later admitted that he went through a two-hour ritual of grooming before he went out, shaving, showering, and selecting his clothes so he would appear "perfect." In addition he was preoccupied with certain "superstitions," such as avoiding a particular building on campus because it was "unlucky," or always lining up his pencils and papers in a certain way when he was preparing his lectures.

Christopher, who was diagnosed as suffering from obsessive-compulsive disorder, was afflicted with obsessions, or recurrent ideas that are not experienced as being voluntarily produced, but rather as thoughts that invade the consciousness and that are often perceived by the patient as senseless. He showed clear signs of compulsions—repetitive behavior patterns performed according to certain rules that served no useful function, were not pleasurable, and were perceived as senseless.

Every disease has its symptoms. We know we have a cold because of the runny nose, the fever, the headache, or the persistent cough. Doctors decide to take certain tests based on hearing and seeing a patient's symptoms. Since we have now established that mental illness can be looked at in the same way as physical illness, it too has specific manifestations. While we will be examining in later chapters of this book the symptoms particular to certain disorders, it is necessary to first provide this overview of the types of behavioral irregularities that can mark a mental imbalance.

The symptoms of mental illness are caused by both external and internal forces. They may seem perplexing and unusual, but they usually have their causes and meanings. They represent the patient's way of maintaining his or her emotional equilibrium. At first glance, a person who has to dress in a certain order each day may appear to be performing a pointless ritual, but in actuality, this can be the way an obsessive-compulsive patient relieves some of his ever-present anxiety.

It would be impossible to list all the symptoms of emotional illness in this chapter—that would take another book to do adequately—but we should see what some of the main manifestations are.

SOMATIC SYMPTOMS

These are the physical symptoms of mental illness, which are not caused by a disease but are still not under the patient's voluntary control. They can include sensations of extreme pain, paralysis or hypochondriasis (in which a person believes he suffers from a serious illness when he is actually in good health). The symptoms may often be linked to a specific reaction to the external world. The term "hysteria," now commonly called *conversion disorder*, is used to describe this phenomena. People can become hysterically deaf to avoid hearing something feared or forbidden. Hysterical paralysis, which is often seen in the armed forces, may start as a way of avoiding a specific activity, such as fighting in a war. One patient who was traumatized by his experiences in World War II found he could no longer face the world. Because he could not deal with holding down a job and supporting his family, even though he knew he was expected by society to do so, he developed paralysis of the legs and truly could not walk until years of intensive therapy cleared up the underlying problems.

PSYCHOLOGICAL SYMPTOMS
Disturbances of Mood, Feeling, Emotion

Anxiety is one of the most common emotional symptoms. It is a very unpleasant sensation of uneasiness, apprehension, or fear stemming from the belief that some type of danger lies "out there," even when no such threat exists. There are different degrees of anxiety, and many of us have experienced some minor form of this emotion at some time. *Free-floating anxiety* is severe, and persistent. It is typically found in mental problems classified as anxiety disorders and can develop into a state known as panic. *Agitation*, which can also appear in anxiety disorders, is a state of restlessness and uneasiness often marked by actions such as pacing or constant nail-biting and mental upset. The body may visibly shake, because physiological effects of anxiety affect the muscular system. *Tension* involves tautness, restlessness, and a feeling of dread.

Panic is an acute attack of anxiety of such overwhelming proportions that it can seriously disrupt daily life. It affects the body and mind and is best described as a reaction to terror that has no source. The word comes from *Pan*, the Greek god who would appear without warning to travelers in the woods, causing "panic."

Normal anxiety is familiar to all of us. It is not a mental problem, because the source of the anxiety is real. The man who becomes fearful because he has lost his job and may not be able to support his family is usually not suffering from an anxiety-related disorder. He is simply reacting appropriately to a stressful situation.

Depression, probably the most common symptom of affective (mood) disturbances, is a feeling of sadness, loneliness, or hopelessness. It is typically found in major depressive disorder and manic-depression (bipolar disorder). It is not the same as grief, where again, the depression corresponds to a real external loss, such as the death of a loved one. However, if the depression over this type of incident continues for an inappropriate length of time, there may also be underlying psychological problems.

Euphoria is an exaggerated sense of happiness not consistent with reality. It is the opposite extreme from depression, and can also signal a serious mental disorder. The person who sleeps only two hours a night for several weeks, loudly boasting that he or she has developed a plan to save the world from all its problems, is not acting rationally, no matter how much singing or dancing around with joy he or she exhibits. Euphoria is most commonly found in manic-depression and in certain organic mental disorders (physical damage to the brain or brain diseases such as senility). The abuse of drugs such as cocaine or amphetamines may also be the cause.

As with anxiety, euphoria may be divided into degrees. *Elation* is noticeable euphoria accompanied by increased physical activity. *Exaltation* is intense euphoria coupled with grandiose feelings, such as the belief that one can fly. *Ecstasy* is a feeling of intense but tranquil euphoria. Religious obsessions are often a part of this emotion. Once again, however, the normal euphoria we may feel when we have received a promotion at work, or when the person we love reciprocates that affection, is the natural emotion of joy and happiness. It has a real external cause and is not an illness.

Apathy is the lack of feeling, emotion, interest or concern about anything. It may be a symptom of depressive illness. *Inappropriateness* is a reaction that is the opposite to what one would expect in a situation. It is exemplified by the person who laughs or giggles upon receiving bad news, and is observed frequently in persons with schizophrenic disorders. *Ambivalence* is a state where the patient has conflicting feelings, such as love and hate, for the same person or object. It is found in many emotional disorders, but particularly in depressive and obsessive-compulsive disorders, and is one of the symptoms of schizophrenia.

Hostility is anger or antagonism in both thought and behavior. It is related to aggression, and violent behavior is the behavioral expression of extreme hostility. In depressive illness, unexpressed and internalized hostility may be an underlying factor.

Depersonalization is the sensation of unreality, strangeness, or altered identity. The patient does not seem "right" to himself for some reason. While it is found in schizophrenia and manic-depressive disorders, it can crop up in healthy people who have suffered from extreme exhaustion or some kind of shock.

Derealization is the feeling that the environment has changed and accompanies mood swings from depression to elation. It is often found in a disease known as cyclothymic disorder, a mood-swing illness lasting for more than two years but not of enough severity to be classed as a major depressive or bipolar illness. It also appears in depersonalization disorders.

Disturbances of Memory

Amnesia is a pathological loss of memory, which may be caused by a head injury, or by certain dissociative psychiatric disorders, such as psychogenic amnesia. It can involve many types of memory alterations, including a loss of memory of events occurring after a specific time, or before a specific time. A *fugue state* is a flight from the *immediate* environment, where one cannot remember what is happening or has just happened.

Hypermnesia is an abnormally vivid or complete memory, or the reawakening of forgotten memories. It is found in both normal people and those who have certain manic or paranoid illnesses.

Paramnesia is a distortion or falsification of memory in which the person confuses reality and fantasy, including the remembrance of scenes and incidents that were never experienced. One patient described to his doctor in detail the pride he felt when he delivered the valedictorian's address to his high school graduating class. Not only was he not the class valedictorian, he had never graduated from high school.

Disturbances of Consciousness

Confusion is disorientation with respect to time, place or person and is commonly found in people with organic mental disorders. *Clouding of consciousness* is a state where information cannot be retained or absorbed and can also accompany senility or other organic disorders. *Dream state,* also known as twilight state, is a period where the person becomes unaware of reality and can behave violently or deviate from his or her usual behavior patterns. This condition can be caused by the use of certain drugs, particularly those similar to atropine, or it can be found in dissociative and convulsive disorders.

Delirium is a disturbance of mood, memory, orientation, and consciousness. The delirious patient may be confused, disoriented, restless, and very excited, unable to fall asleep, and incapable of carrying out any purposeful mental activity. Illusions and hallucinations can occur, and this symptom is often seen with the abuse of alcohol and/or drugs, and in serious infectious diseases. *Coma* is a state of extreme unconsciousness, found in certain organic disorders and in the stuporous form of catatonic schizophrenia. *Catatonia* is marked by a decrease in the person's reactions to his own environment, a reduction in movement and activity, and often the absence of speech. The patient may sit motionless for hours or even days in a single position. *Deterioration* or *dementia* is the progressive loss of both emotional and intellectual functions, found most often in Alzheimer's disease and other forms of senility. Reversible deterioration can occur in the schizophrenic.

Disturbances of Perception

Illusions are misinterpretations of experiences involving the senses, usually sight or hearing. They are often quite normal. One example of an optical illusion is the way heat waves shimmering on a road resemble pools of water. An auditory illusion may be the way the wind can sound like the cry of a human voice. Illusions can also appear during withdrawal from alcohol addiction.

Hallucinations are not as normal, because there is no external cause for the false perception of the senses. They occur in substance-abuse disorders caused by alcohol, cocaine, or hallucinogens such as LSD, peyote, or mescaline. They are also found in schizophrenics and manics.

Disturbances of Speech

Ecolalia is the repetition of the phrases or words of another person. It is found in organic illnesses as well as in schizophrenia. Other problems with verbal behavior can include extremely rapid speech, incoherent speech, or excessive talking.

Disturbances of Motor Behavior

The symptoms in this category include excessive movements, slow movements or lack of movement (including not moving from whatever position one has been placed in), trance-like states, unusual postures, strange mannerisms such as excessive blinking, constant repetition of one particular type of activity such as snapping one's fingers, or ritualistic motions designed to ward off some imaginary fear or threatening person. In William Wharton's book *Birdy*, the main character, shocked by his war experiences, is placed in a mental ward because he will not communicate and sits all day perched in a corner (mimicking the posture of birds, which were his hobby and obsession throughout youth).

Disturbances of Thought

Thought is the exercise of our powers of judgment, conception, and discrimination, and falls prey to many symptomatic disorders. *Fantasy* is daydreaming, the mental construction of a series of pictures or events. It may express unconscious conflicts, gratify otherwise unobtainable wishes, or provide a partial or total escape from reality. *Obsessions* are recurrent and persistent ideas, images, thoughts, or impulses that remain in the conscious mind despite their seeming pointlessness. A person who constantly visualizes coffins has an obsession. This symptom is typically found in obsessive-compulsive illness. *Phobias* are extreme and irrational fears of specific objects, activities or situations. Examples include the fear of heights, closed spaces, open spaces, animals, or dirt.

Delusions are false beliefs that are not consistent with reality or the person's intellect. They can include the conviction that one is being controlled by alien thoughts circulating through the air, or that one has been singled out for harassment or attack. Self-accusatory delusions exist when persons feel they are responsible for some harm they have had no part in, or believe that even their normal behavior is somehow "wrong."

Blocking is difficulty in remembering or understanding a section of thought or speech because of conscious emotional forces. For instance, a schizophrenic may stop talking, or block, because he is now listening to an imaginary voice, or because of his own conflicting reactions to what he is saying.

Incoherence is disorderly, illogical thought, which sometimes comes out as garbled speech. *Flight of ideas* is skipping from one thought to another in quick succession, without ever reaching the goal of the conversation. It is frequently observed in manic episodes, as well as with the abuse of certain recreational drugs such as cocaine or LSD.

Disturbances of Attention

These symptoms can include a decrease in attention, a fluctuation of attention even when the person tries to apply himself, a blunting of attention (which is extreme inattention, so that even a loud noise occurring right next to the person will not elicit a response), and increased attention or hyperprosexia, which is unusual concentration, normally given to details of personal significance.

While we have examined only a partial list, a complete knowledge of symptoms such as these is vital to the physician so that the patient's underlying illness or mental status can be determined. Only then can a working diagnosis and treatment program begin. The right type of therapy and/or drugs must be used if the patient is to be helped. For example, a schizophrenic will not usually show much improvement if placed only on antidepressant medication. Therefore, if a person with schizophrenia is admitted to the hospital and at the time is exhibiting only symptoms of depression, the physician, through careful questioning and examination, must eventually come to the correct conclusion in order to help the patient. Unfortunately, many disorders can masquerade as others, or a less serious problem may be covering up something more profound. Extensive questioning and examination of the person's behavior is necessary to find the underlying illness—the one that must be tackled if complete recovery is the goal.

CHAPTER FOUR

The Many Forms of Treatment

Millie knew there was something wrong with her. She couldn't seem to get out of bed in the morning, had lost interest in herself and her family, and frequently contemplated suicide. She realized she was profoundly depressed, but she couldn't figure out why. Her marriage was happy and sound, her children were well-behaved and loving—everything seemed so perfect. Yet inside her was a storm of blackness, making her ache night and day with a non-specific grief. When her sister mentioned seeing a psychiatrist, Millie became more distraught than shocked. She didn't want to go regularly to a doctor for years and years who might never even get to the root of the problem. She didn't understand how a therapist could help her out of this depression. To her, only a "real" doctor was worth going to—he took appropriate tests, found out what was wrong, and prescribed treatment that made you better. "Shrinks," in her view, just groped in the dark.

Millie's opinion of the science of psychiatry is more typical than not. It is also inaccurate. Investigators of the mind are becoming increasingly precise in diagnosis and treatment, and a person has many options. Sitting and talking for years with an analyst is by no means the only form of therapy.

The First Visit
Most people don't know what to expect the first time they see a therapist. Actually, they will be put through an extensive "interview" in which the doctor gathers information about:

• The present complaint and any symptoms related to it.
• Any history connected to the present problem (i.e., whether the problem has happened before).
• If there is a history, how the patient adjusted to the symptoms and his environment in the past.

- The patient's family and marital history.
- The patient's educational, social, and occupational background.
- Medical history (including information from the patient's doctors).

A routine physical and neurological examination is an essential part of this first step in the psychiatric process. This ensures that no organic disease such as hyperthyroidism or hypoglycemia is causing the symptoms.

The patient is sometimes given various psychological tests to determine the nature of the symptoms and disorder. In the case of serious illness, family members are also interviewed.

The doctor then decides how to treat the patient, choosing from the many different approaches to therapy that are used today—including pharmacotherapy or chemotherapy, which is based on the assumption that a drug program is effective in treating psychiatric disorders because of its action on the central nervous system (CNS)—the brain and spinal cord. This implies that at least some ailments are caused or exacerbated by defective functioning of the CNS.

Although the accent in this book is on chemical therapy, this therapy should be used in combination with some other form of treatment. For that reason, a brief explanation of the major treatment options is necessary. It is also important to remember that most modern therapists use a combination of treatment methods and may tailor their programs to suit the needs of the individual patient.

TYPES OF THERAPY

Before discussing the different forms of therapy, a brief description of some relevant terms concerning the various types of mental disorders is necessary. The word *neurosis,* coined by the Englishman William Cullen in 1769, was used at that time to refer to disordered sensations of the nervous system. Today, the term "neurotic," although used loosely by the general public to refer to almost every type of unusual or maladaptive behavior, actually has a specific meaning. It refers to those disorders in which inner psychological conflict, the anxiety it causes, and the resulting efforts of the person to build defenses in order to control the anxiety, are thought to be central in causing the behavioral abnormality. However, since certain experts believed this model was "too theoretical," the authors of the *DSM-III* removed the term "neuroses" as a general category, and instead developed new categories such as anxiety or somatoform disorders. Psychosis, on the other hand, is a term still widely in use, and refers to severe psychological problems that involve a loss of contact with reality and gross personality distortions. Paranoid disorders and schizophrenia fall into this category. Neurosis is certainly the less severe of the two, and most neurotic patients recover from their symptoms and never develop any kind of psychoses.

Individual Psychotherapy

This is a process by which a person who wants to relieve symptoms or resolve problems in living (or who is just seeking personal growth) decides to talk about and explore these questions with a therapist in a prescribed way. The doctor may decide to deal with past causes of a problem, offer strategies for more healthy interactions with the environment and outside stressors, use hypnosis, or employ a variety of techniques to help the patient and relieve the disturbing symptoms of a disorder, if one exists.

Patients with neurotic disorders often improve a great deal following short periods of verbal or behavioral psychotherapy, and many neurotic patients who do not respond to therapy do react positively to some of the various psychoactive drugs. Other studies show that the combination of psychotherapy and antidepressants results in significant improvement in people with affective disorders (depression, manic-depression—see Chapter Seven). Many schizophrenics are treated with antipsychotic drugs and supportive therapy (a type of treatment where the patient's strengths and assets are pointed out and developed).

Group Psychotherapy

This is the application of therapeutic techniques to a group, and includes as part of the treatment the interactions between members of the group as well as their interactions with the therapist. Groups are usually composed of one therapist and six to eight patients, who may or may not have similarities in their backgrounds or symptoms. This category also includes self-help groups such as Alcoholics Anonymous (AA), where the members share a common symptom, though not always the same underlying problem.

Family Therapy

This is a form of group therapy, where the nuclear family is the unit. It has developed over the last three or four decades, and is used where emotional disturbances of individual members are believed to be outgrowths of conflicts within the family.

Adjunctive Therapies

Usually employed in hospital settings, these therapies include activities, such as occupational therapies, group craft projects, homemaking sessions, and therapeutic recreation (volleyball). Expressive therapies are also included here, such as music therapy, dance therapy, art therapy, or workshops in creative writing.

Somatic Therapy

The two major forms of somatic therapy are electroconvulsive therapy (shock therapy) and/or psychosurgery, in which parts of the brain are operated on, according to the problem. These are extreme methods and normally not employed for minor neurotic complaints. Since the introduction of antipsychotic and antidepressant drugs in the late 1950s and early 1960s, the use of electroconvulsive therapy (ECT) as a treatment for schizophrenic disorders has declined, but it is still used for acute affective (mood) disorders such as severe depression. There are many theories about how it works, but no one knows for certain. In ECT, enough electrical current is passed through electrodes attached to both temporal areas of the head to produce a grand mal seizure (as in epilepsy). A series of these treatments is usually given—from six to twelve being the average.

The popular media has sometimes used ECT as a symbol of the horror that takes place in mental hospitals, but the issue is not so clear-cut. ECT is recommended in cases of:

- severe depression, where the risk of suicide is high, the patient is not eating or drinking enough to sustain life, and the use of drugs is too risky or will take too long;
- severe psychosis, where the safety of the patient or those around him is threatened by his behavior;
- severe catatonia, which does not respond to any other form of treatment because the doctor cannot communicate with the patient;
- severe mania, where the use of drugs entails a great risk, as when a medical problem (such as a recent heart attack) requires prompt treatment of the over-excited state, and makes many drugs unacceptable.

Psychosurgery, the other image of horror, is now rarely employed. Most people think of the term "lobotomy" when such surgery is mentioned, although in reality there are many different types. Lobotomies, the most extreme form, have almost disappeared from use. Only people with crippling mental disorders who have not responded at all to treatment and whose chance of recovery is very poor are candidates for this extreme type of therapy. More than 50% of these people show improvement after the surgery, although some get worse.

Behavior Therapy

This is a broad category that defines all types of therapy based on the principle that a person's behavior is a result of what has been learned. It can be loosely defined as the modification of a person's responses to a situation through the application of techniques designed to reinforce or change those responses. The treatment is geared toward removing inappropriate behavior (and symptoms) and toward learning new, more productive patterns of reaction.

Humanistic Therapy

This newer form of therapy is hard to define. It is a term used to describe the thinking of some doctors who react against traditional psychoanalysis and behavior therapy. They feel that a person's choices, even if eccentric, are a manifestation of his own free will. The emphasis here is on the identification and acceptance of one's needs and personal responsibility for meeting them by selecting effective and non-harmful strategies. These therapists feel that many symptoms are caused by a person's evasion of responsibility for his own choices.

This type of treatment is seen by many as unscientific, although it has become very popular. It presents the idea that every person is unique, and therefore personal dignity must not be insulted by the attempts of others to categorize, label or make generalizations about human character and/or behavior.

As a leading psychiatrist recently pointed out, the fact that there is some disagreement among therapists does not show the science is weak, but strong, creative, and adaptable. Each patient is an individual, and certain types of treatment work better for some than others. It is fortunate for us all that there are now many choices.

CHAPTER FIVE

When Do Drugs Help?

Ryan, the anxious writer mentioned at the beginning of the book, eventually worked out his problems in therapy. But the relief for his immediate symptoms—the panic attacks that were preventing him from working or enjoying life—came from the medication prescribed by his psychiatrist.

Among all the different types of therapy, the quickest and easiest way of relieving symptoms is through the use of drugs. But chemical treatment is not effective in the management of every psychological disorder. It is most beneficial for certain types of illnesses. This chapter is designed to give an introductory overview of all the disorders treated with medication, and following chapters will then explore the major ones in greater detail.

Anxiety Disorders

In this group, the feeling of anxiety is either the main problem (as in panic disorder and generalized anxiety disorder), or is the sensation experienced by the person when he or she attempts to overcome the symptoms (i.e., confronting the dreaded object or situation in a phobic disorder, or resisting the obsessions and compulsions in obsessive-compulsive disorder). The medications mainly used here are antianxiety agents such as benzodiazepines, or a new drug, buspirone. If symptoms of depression accompany the anxiety, antidepressants may be added to the treatment program.

Somatoform Disorders

The features that mark this group are physical symptoms, such as paralysis of a limb. These symptoms suggest an organic illness, except that medical testing shows that nothing is wrong and there is strong evidence in the person's behavior to suggest that the symptoms are somehow linked to psychological factors or conflicts. The symptoms are not under the person's voluntary control; the inability to walk is valid as far as the patient is concerned—he cannot get up and run around even if he desperately wants to. Antianxiety and antidepressant drugs are used in the treatment of these disorders.

Psychosomatic Disorders

Psychosomatic gastrointestinal reactions. Almost everyone is aware of the relationship between the emotions and digestion. Depressed people often eat more. Anxious people may avoid food for days. It is thought that food may be associated with feelings of security, attention, and love. Various types of psychosomatic problems are associated with eating, digesting, and eliminating food, such as *anorexia nervosa* (marked by a severe and prolonged refusal to eat) or obesity (which can be caused by depression). Anorexia is often treated with antidepressant drugs, and obesity can be treated with amphetamine-like compounds for a short period of time. When depression accompanies the disorder, as with obesity or bulimia (binge-eating), antidepressants may be used.

Psychosomatic musculoskeletal disorders, such as tension headaches, are often helped by antianxiety and/or antidepressant drugs.

Psychosomatic respiratory disorders, in which emotions such as hostility, anxiety, fear, or excitement lead to disturbances in breathing, can be treated with antianxiety and antidepressant medications.

Psychosexual Disorders

With psychosexual disorders, a person's sexual behavior in some way significantly deviates from the norm. Among the numerous types of problematic sexual behavior included in this category, only one is treated with medication, and that is ego-dystonic homosexuality. Homosexuality, as such, is no longer considered deviant or a psychiatric problem, but rather the choice to follow an alternate life-style. Ego-dystonic homosexuality, in which the person does not want to follow this life-style and really would like to be heterosexual, or is not adjusting to his or her homosexuality, is considered a problem. Antianxiety agents or antidepressants have been prescribed for the anxiety and/or depression that can accompany this disorder.

Affective (Mood) Disorders

The term "affective disorder" is a general one and refers to a mental problem in which the fundamental disturbance lies in the mood of the person—which can reach psychotic proportions. The mood changes to depression, elation, or back and forth between the two—differ from normal "ups" and "downs" chiefly in their severity and duration. Mood changes may happen with no apparent outside cause, may be out of proportion to the outside cause, or may persist too long after the outside cause has occurred.

In recent years, a great deal of research has gone into examining the reasons and possible treatment for such disorders. Improvements have been made in various drug therapies, including the use of tricyclic antidepressants (TCAs), monoamine oxidase inhibitors (MAOIs), lithium, and newer antidepressant agents.

Personality Disorders

These are marked by their lifelong nature, and the person's often self-defeating behavior can make it impossible in many cases for him to lead a normal life. These problems can be grouped into three basic categories:

- The type of person who appears strange or very eccentric, and may be suffering from either paranoid or schizophrenic-like diseases. There may be an inability to relate to others in a sincere or caring way, and/or disturbances in speech, thought, or behavior. However, these patients are not ill enough to be classified as schizophrenic.
- People who exhibit overly dramatic, emotional, or erratic behavior.
- People who appear anxious or afraid.

Usually, the symptoms of personality disorders do not seem to bother the patient to any great degree, so various types of non-chemical therapy may be enough for treatment. However, if anxiety or depression is present, antianxiety, antidepressant, or antipsychotic medications may also be used.

Substance-Use Disorders

These disorders involve the abuse of harmful drugs, such as cocaine, heroin, alcohol, etc. The withdrawal from many of these drugs requires medication to help the patient through difficult periods. During the detoxification period from drugs such as cocaine, amphetamines, and hallucinogens (e.g., LSD), certain other drugs are carefully prescribed. These include benzodiazepine tranquilizers such as chlordiazepoxide (Librium), diazepam (Valium), or barbiturates such as phenobarbital. They are continued for several days after the patient has stopped using the harmful drugs. Clonidine (Catapres), an antihypertensive agent, has been used with some success in withdrawing people from methadone.

Alcoholism is a special type of substance-use disorder that deserves more in-depth examination, mainly because of its frequent appearance in the population. By the definition of the World Health Organization, alcoholics are those excessive drinkers whose dependence on drinking has reached such a degree that it causes a noticeable mental disturbance, or interferes with their physical and mental health, their social relationships, and their overall functioning in life.

It is hard to say how many people in this country are alcoholics. Of course, not everyone who gets drunk from time to time can be considered one. Of the estimated 120 million people in the U.S. who drink, about nine or ten million could be thought of as alcohol-dependent. There are about five to six times as many male problem-drinkers as females.

There are often a number of underlying emotional problems that can contribute to a person becoming an alcoholic—the chief ones involving depression or some type of anxiety, which is quieted by drinking to excess. For example, Fred, a publishing executive, suddenly lost his job and was unable to find a comparable one. He had suffered through a childhood of abuse at the hands of his religiously fanatic father, which had made him deeply fearful and insecure. But his rapid climb in the business world has boosted his ravaged ego, and so no symptoms appeared until his career collapsed. He then began having severe anxiety attacks, found he was even unable to drive a car, and couldn't face job interviews. He started to drink heavily. Although he eventually found a good position, the constant, heavy drinking continued. He entered a clinic only after he had lost his family and his new job.

Alcohol withdrawal is handled with a combination of drugs. Librium (chlordiazepoxide) is given in fairly large doses for several days before being tapered down and discontinued; or Valium (diazepam) may be employed instead. If a withdrawal seizure (convulsion) is anticipated, an anticonvulsant drug such as Dilantin (phenytoin) may be added, but most people do not need to be maintained on anticonvulsant drugs. For treatment of the chronic mental disorders that accompany alcoholism, antidepressants are used to relieve the "blues." When Librium and Valium are used for withdrawal, they must be prescribed with caution and for only a short period of time, or the alcoholic can become dependent on these drugs instead of alcohol.

There are other medications that were once more commonly employed in the management of alcoholism than they are today. One such drug is disulfiram (Antabuse) which was developed in 1948. The patient becomes violently ill, with effects such as nausea, headaches, and weakness, if he drinks alcohol in any form while taking the drug. Its effects wear off in a few days after use is discontinued, and people must be in good health to take it. Many people object to this type of behavior modification treatment, known as aversion therapy.

The severe alcoholic is often hospitalized. Psychotherapy, group therapy, and support organizations such as Alcoholics Anonymous (AA) are used to help the heavy drinker cope with his underlying problems and get him off alcohol. There is a growing amount of evidence to show that the tendency toward alcoholism may be inherited, but in any event it is certainly one of this country's major concerns. In fact, it is one of the four main health problems in America (the others are mental disorders, cardiovascular disease, and cancer).

Adjustment Disorders

These problems occur when an outside event, such as the death of a loved one, causes an extreme reaction, such as severe anxiety or prolonged (over a year) depression. In some cases, antianxiety or antidepressive drugs are used, especially if the symptoms disrupt the patient's social and business life.

Schizophrenic Disorders

This term covers a wide group of problems. They are usually of psychotic proportion, and marked by problems with communication, language, thought, perception, mood, and behavior that lasts longer than six months. Some people experience a schizophrenic episode only once in their lives, while many suffer from this problem from childhood through old age. The medications prescribed in these cases include mainly antipsychotic agents. Intramuscular injection of a long-acting phenothiazine (an antipsychotic) such as Prolixin (fluphenazine) may be used for noncompliant patients, or until the patient becomes more cooperative toward other forms of treatment. Some patients also prefer receiving an injection once every two weeks, rather than having to take oral medication on a daily basis.

Paranoid Disorders

These disorders are marked by hyperalertness, suspiciousness, delusions, and distortions of reality. The paranoid patient blames others or society for his problems, and his emotions can reach psychotic proportions. People with paranoid disorders are mainly using the psychological defense mechanism of *projection*, in which they attribute to other persons or objects the thoughts, feelings, motives, or hopes that really belong to them, but which for some reason they cannot accept. Various antipsychotic drugs can help the patient tone down these delusions and assist in his adaptation back into society.

Organic Mental Disorders

Brain damage or disease can cause organic mental disorders (Alzheimer's disease, brain tumors, accidents). Phenothiazines may be used for the agitation that can accompany senility; in some of these cases, antidepressants or antianxiety agents are prescribed. Small doses are usually recommended, because patients with brain problems can be very sensitive to the effects of these medications.

Although we will be examining both the diseases and drugs in greater detail, it is important to have a relative "feel" for the subject at this point, so certain terms and conditions are not mysterious. This field need not seem frightening and complex. As more is learned, things are becoming much clearer, and cures far more common.

CHAPTER SIX

Anxiety and Anxiety Disorders

Recently, a young woman wrote the following letter to a medical columnist in a major local newspaper:

"Since I was a child, I experienced episodes of panic. I would feel as though I was suffocating, that my heart was going to burst, or that I would faint—all from some fear I couldn't understand. I had no idea why I had these feelings. I was at first sure they were signs of some terrible illness, but no doctor could find anything wrong with me. Several times I found myself in a hospital emergency room where I would be given a tranquilizing injection and told to 'calm down.' These attacks could strike as many as three or four times a day. I used to wake up sweating, screaming, or gasping for air.

"Believe it or not, I managed to function through all this. I was never without a job, and I made excellent money. I have had comfortable, long-term relationships with men, close relationships with family members, and a generally active social life. However, when I turned 25, I could no longer tolerate these disabling episodes. They were becoming more intense and more frequent. I didn't want to see a psychiatrist for fear I'd be branded 'crazy' but I now knew it was my only chance to recover. I was lucky in that I found a wonderful analyst on the first try. It took a while, but she and I worked together, using regular therapy and some medication—a drug called Xanax—and eventually those dreadful episodes stopped completely. I now believe that it is essential for people with this problem to see someone trained in the field of psychology."

The columnist answered:

"What you've described is called anxiety, or panic attacks. More than one million Americans suffer from them. Often these attacks include a problem known as agoraphobia, which limits a person's movements only to comfortable surroundings. Some authorities say that these out-of-the-blue attacks are caused by a biochemical abnormality of the nervous system, which may be inherited. Drug therapy has been found to be very useful in treating this problem."

ANXIETY

Anxiety, in the psychiatric sense, is not like simple nervousness. The jitters we may experience before going to an important interview or speaking in front of a large group of people are often natural feelings, and easily overcome. Clinical anxiety is an overpowering sensation of fear, agitation, or dread, which can disrupt lives and limit activity. When it is severe or prolonged, it becomes highly distressing and must be treated. In fact, the symptoms of anxiety-related problems are so upsetting that most people are unable to tolerate them for any extended length of time and so do seek help.

Anxiety is similar to fear, and comes from within the personality in response to some type of threat, known or unknown. It produces changes in the body itself—some physical processes are stimulated while others are inhibited. This happens because the body reacts instinctively to a threatening situation by alerting the mind and gearing up for vigorous activity. This reaction is known as the "fight or flight response" and it helps us in many ways when we are faced with a real threat. Unfortunately, the body doesn't know when the fear is caused by a real external problem and when it is caused by psychological stress, so the same response is invoked either way.

Our bodies react in three major ways to stress. First, the hormone epinephrine (Adrenalin) is secreted by the central nervous system and causes the physical responses of anxiety. The mental manifestation of this action is the sensation of fear and discomfort. Meanwhile, in the body, the heart rate is affected, causing rapid beating or palpitations. There is usually an increase in blood pressure, and premature contractions of the heart. Sometimes the cardiovascular system is slowed down, and a person can feel faint or dizzy. The salivary glands are inhibited, which causes "dry mouth." There may be a foul taste in the mouth, nausea, vomiting, cramps, loss of appetite, "butterflies" in the stomach, diarrhea, or constipation. The person may suffer from rapid breathing, constant sighing, or hyperventilation. There may be increased urination, pelvic pain, frigidity, or impotence. Sweating or flushing may occur, along with trembling muscles (often first seen in the lips), dilation of the nostrils, tension headaches, constriction in the back of the neck, a quiver in the voice, arthritis-like pains, and various other muscle and joint disturbances.

All of these physical changes are caused by the body's reaction to anxiety. If you were being chased down a dark street, many of these reactions would come to your aid in helping you to get away. However, when there is no real physical threat, the body reactions triggered by anxiety only serve to make a person feel extremely uncomfortable.

Cause and Treatment

Anxiety disorders can be triggered by a conflict between the external world and the personality, such as having to work at an unfulfilling, dull job when a person is highly motivated and creative. They may also be caused by a conflict between a person's instinctual drives and the censoring forces against them, such as when a housewife wants to go back to work in an office and her family doesn't want her to do so. The tension created by two conflicting desires (i.e., the need to leave a spouse versus the fear of doing so) can also result in anxiety. If the anxiety becomes severe, the person is compelled to do something about it, such as move around nervously or, too often, drink alcohol. Many people with anxiety disorders lean toward alcoholism if they are not treated properly.

Many researchers today believe that a predisposition to panic disorder may run in families, and be caused by a brain chemical imbalance affecting the neurotransmitter norepinephrine, which helps regulate physiological arousal. The area of the brain most often mentioned in these studies is the *locus ceruleus*, a structure located deep in the brain that seems to control emotional responses as well as certain involuntary functions. The cells in this area are rich in norepinephrine. The theory is that people with panic disorder have some basic metabolic defect that results in an over-release of norepinephrine in the locus ceruleus, causing the emotional and physical changes that accompany this type of anxiety disorder. The female hormone progesterone, released during the latter part of the menstrual cycle, may also have some effect on the ailment, but more research is needed before any theories can be offered.

The rule for seeking treatment is simple: If the anxiety has a real cause and lasts for a short period of time, it is usually an understandable and normal reaction; if it is triggered for no reason and is persistent and severe, there is a psychological problem. When someone has an anxiety disorder, he may know there is no reason for his feelings of fear, but he is still unable to make them go away. Only professional treatment can do that.

The treatment for anxiety-related problems involves some type of therapy (see Chapter Four), which often includes life-changing strategies. Careful personal planning can help—disorganization can cause feelings of panic. Radical steps such as entering a therapeutic program, finding a new job, leaving a partner, changing the environment, or putting more emphasis on enjoyable hobbies and physical exercise can all release the tension.

While therapy is essential when a person suffers from severe anxiety, that therapy may be threatened by the very symptoms of the problem. Overly fearful, nervous people may find it difficult to communicate or even to face their problems because this causes more anxiety. The solution to this dilemma has come in the form of antianxiety medications.

These drugs can remove the crippling symptoms of the disorder, providing a tremendous aid to successful therapy.

ANXIETY DISORDERS

Anxiety and depression are two of the most common symptoms seen by psychiatrists. As much as four percent of the population experiences anxiety as a disorder at one time or another. There are several different types of anxiety disorders, but in all cases anxiety is either the main disturbance, or it comes as a result of trying to cope with the symptoms of another type of problem. An example is when a person with a phobic fear of heights is forced to face the fear (i.e., look over the top of a high building), and anxiety ensues.

Phobic Disorder

Some people suffer from persistent, irrational fears of a specific object, activity, or situation, and will avoid facing these things at all costs. The person may know that the fear is unfounded, but cannot help the reaction. A famous boxer who feared no man in the ring and was almost immune to pain could not ride in elevators because of his claustrophobia, or fear of enclosed spaces.

Kathleen, an attorney in her late thirties, sought psychiatric help for her intense fear of thunderstorms. Although she had suffered from this phobia since she was a child, its severity had increased during recent years, to the point where if she heard a thunderstorm was expected by the end of the week, her dread would begin to mount until that time. She knew the fear was irrational, but that knowledge did not help her. During a storm, she would make sure someone else was with her, and move to a part of the house where she could not see the lightning should it occur.

Sixty percent of all phobic patients suffer from a form of the disease known as *agoraphobia,* more commonly found in women. Here there is a fear of being alone, or in public places from which escape may be difficult or help not available if the person suddenly becomes ill. Normal activities are limited to a greater degree as this fear begins to dominate the person's life. Many sufferers cannot even leave their homes. Mary, a 31-year-old housewife, could not step over the threshold of her front door without experiencing a crippling sense of panic. The most common situations that agoraphobics avoid are being in crowds (i.e., busy streets or large stores), in tunnels, or on bridges, elevators, or public transportation. People with this type of phobia can also suffer from extreme depression.

Social phobics avoid situations where they could be judged by others, such as meetings, parties, conventions, or any type of public speaking. One talented young man turned down a promotion because it involved giving speeches to small groups of people.

Simple phobias involve such things as the fear of certain animals, the fear of enclosed spaces (claustrophobia), and the fear of heights (acrophobia). There are many different types of simple phobias—people have been known to be deathly afraid of loud noises, infants, or even restaurants. The choice of phobia often represents some underlying conflict about a desire or impulse. The person who is afraid of dirt may really want to be soiled, or to do "dirty things."

Some form of psychotherapy is used for all types of phobias. To relieve the alarming symptoms as quickly as possible, antianxiety drugs are often prescribed. The medication can serve a dual purpose in these cases. First, it relieves the anxiety and enables the person to face and discuss the underlying problems with the therapist. Second, it can help the person get through the fearful experience, allowing him to see that it is not as threatening as he first thought it would be. Antidepressants may then be used for maintenance therapy, if needed.

Panic Disorders

An increasing number of people in our society are suffering from panic attacks, as did the young woman who wrote to the newspaper. These spells can occur at unpredictable times, although certain situations, such as driving a car, can bring them on. People with this problem suffer from the sudden onslaught of intense apprehension, fear or terror, which is often accompanied by a sense of impending doom. There may also be fear between the attacks (which can last anywhere from a few minutes to a few hours)—mainly of suffering from another such spell. During the attack itself, the person may feel like he is dying or "going crazy."

When treating panic attacks, the doctor must first rule out certain physical ailments that can cause the same type of symptoms. Mitral valve prolapse (a poorly functioning valve in the heart), hypoglycemia (low blood sugar), tumors in the central nervous system, or hyperthyroidism (an overactive thyroid) could all be responsible.

These attacks may happen only once—or during one period of a person's life—or they can become chronic. They may also be precursors of other psychiatric problems such as schizophrenia or major depressive illness.

Treatment of these spells involves therapy coupled with medication. Antidepressant drugs are tried first, then antianxiety agents if they are needed. When depression appears with the anxiety, antidepressants are also used. In most cases, the antianxiety agents are effective and do significantly reduce the symptoms. One in particular, a drug called alprazolam (Xanax), which appears to have a mild antidepressant effect along with calming anxiety, has been found to virtually eliminate the panic attacks.

Generalized Anxiety Disorder

This illness is treated in the same way as panic disorder. Here there is a chronic (at least one month), general feeling of anxiety. The symptoms are shakiness, trembling, tenseness, restlessness, sweating, a pounding heart, dry mouth, dizziness, tingling in the hands or feet, frequent urination, diarrhea, worry, fear, irritability, a lack of concentration, and insomnia. The person may feel like something terrible is about to happen, or can become startled and agitated at the slightest sound.

Many people with generalized anxiety worry about everything, no matter how well things appear to be going. These vague fears and concerns keep them continually upset, uneasy, and discouraged. They have great difficulty making decisions, and worry afterwards about having done the right thing.

Sometimes generalized anxiety is triggered by a specific incident. Michael, a 50-year-old minister, developed these symptoms after learning his wife had been unfaithful. He blamed himself for his failed marriage, yet he was angry at his spouse for deceiving and humiliating him. While he really wanted a divorce, his moral and religious position prevented him from taking this option. He also felt that because his marriage had failed, he had failed the church he so deeply loved. When he finally went for therapy, he complained of lack of sleep because he would stay up at night worrying about his problems. He was unable to think clearly while performing his everyday duties, and he had lost his appetite because of a burning sensation in his stomach. He told his therapist he had always been an insecure and dependent person who found support in the church and in his strong, independent wife. The minister was a man who became overwhelmed when faced with taking charge of his life and solving his problems.

People with generalized anxiety disorders are treated with therapy and antianxiety drugs, which can remove many of their symptoms. Some recover in a relatively short period of time. However, it is essential that they seek help if the anxiety and other symptoms are severe, because such problems as loss of appetite and high stress can take a toll on their physical health.

Obsessive-Compulsive Disorder (OCD)

Obsessions are recurring, persistent ideas, thoughts, images, or impulses, which the person feels invade his consciousness and are not under his control. Attempts are made to ignore or suppress them. These thoughts or images may be repulsive or disturbing in some way. Compulsions are recurrent, seemingly purposeless behavior patterns that are performed according to certain strange rules or in a ritualistic manner. They are often used to relieve feelings of anxiety.

In obsessive-compulsive disorder, people feel compelled to think about something they do not wish to think about or carry out some action against their will. Many of these patients know their behavior is irrational but cannot control it. In compulsive disorders, people feel compelled to perform some act that seems absurd or bizarre to them and which they do not want to perform. This can range from having to make the sign of the cross at certain times of the day to checking ten times an hour to see if the car door is locked. The compulsive act usually brings some relief from the anxiety of not doing the compulsion or of thinking the obsessive thought.

People with OCD may find it hard to make decisions, and can be filled with constant doubt. Their obsessions may be about anything, but the most common themes are violence, contamination, sexuality, and religion. Common compulsions include handwashing rituals that develop as a means of relieving fears about dirt or germs, or arranging items such as furniture in a specific way.

Fleeting obsessions or compulsions are experienced by most of us at some time, but this does not mean we have OCD. Actually, this problem affects less than five percent of all psychiatric patients. When people do have this disorder, intensive therapy, sometimes administered in a hospital, is necessary. Drugs such as antianxiety and antidepressant agents are often used, but they are not as effective here as with other anxiety-related disorders. Newer antidepressants that increase serotonin, such as clomipramine and fluoxetine, are showing improvement in treatment of OCD.

Post-Traumatic Stress Disorder
This problem is the unfortunate result of an extremely upsetting experience, such as being raped or experiencing a similarly violent crime. The outside cause is real and known and would cause anxiety in anyone, but for these people, the nightmare never leaves them. They may have constant recollections of the event (which can intrude on everyday thoughts), recurrent dreams, or the sudden feeling that the event is happening again, even when the threat is long over.

This is a disorder that almost always follows an incident that involves a direct threat to life. The event may be an assault, military combat, a flood or earthquake, a car accident, a fire or plane crash, or some form of torture. The symptoms must last longer than six months to be considered a problem. One of the largest groups of people to suffer from this disorder are those who survived the Nazi death camps. Soldiers who returned from Vietnam—more than other war veterans—were found in many cases to be suffering from this disorder. The treatment again involves therapy and the administration of antianxiety agents.

In all cases of anxiety disorders, the use of certain medications can relieve or erase the painful and crippling symptoms. While they cannot cure the problem—only therapy and a change in perspective can do that—they can make it easier for a person to function on a day-to-day basis while he or she is dealing with the underlying conflicts that originally caused the disorder.

All of us feel nervous from time to time, many fear the loss of a job or mate, and some people feel the compulsion to do certain things that relieve the tension. But when the fear becomes crippling, and the anxiety causes some type of retreat from a normal life, then treatment is needed. Although feelings of anxiety are among the most uncomfortable symptoms of emotional illness, they can be significantly alleviated through the use of the proper medications.

CHAPTER SEVEN

AFFECTIVE (MOOD) DISORDERS: Are You "Up" or "Down"?

Leslie married Sam after knowing him only six weeks, but his remarkable energy and charisma had literally swept her off her feet. He never seemed to need sleep, was always coming up with creative new ideas, and was obviously quite successful, judging by the way he spent money. His optimism and zest for life were infectious, and although he sometimes exhausted her, the excitement he provided made up for it. Sexually he was expert and aggressive, and never seemed to lose interest or energy.

Shortly after their marriage, Leslie came home to find a different Sam. He huddled in the corner of the bed—where he remained—hardly able to speak, crying soundlessly, with no interest in food, sex, or even life. He dropped off to sleep without the slightest provocation, and just wanted to "be left alone." Leslie also found a stack of unpaid bills and found out that Sam was deeply in debt, spending much more money than he made. He kept asking her to forgive him, told her he was worthless, and suggested that if she really loved him she would put him out of his misery by helping him kill himself.

Leslie realized that something was wrong psychologically with her husband, although he denied it. He finally agreed to see a therapist for her sake. The diagnosis was manic-depression, now more commonly called bipolar illness. Sam was suffering from dramatic and recurrent mood swings—from the heights of elation to the depths of depression and back again. His treatment began with therapy and a medication called lithium, which has been shown to prevent recurrences of bipolar symptoms.

Sam stayed in therapy and took the lithium for about six months, during which time his moods were more even. But he began to complain that he had lost his "highs" and stopped the medication. Soon he was in a manic stage again, although this time it reached a degree that frightened his wife. At first he was elated and energetic, but then he became incoherent, enraged over nothing, and spoke to people who weren't there. He spent every penny they had, and then boasted he could "make it back in a minute." He told her that he was on the verge of finding a cure for cancer, and designing a spaceship that could travel to Venus in a matter of hours. When she tried to convince him to see the doctor again, he started to break up the furniture in the house and threatened to kill her. He almost never slept, and moved around constantly. Leslie didn't know what to do.

The situation resolved itself in an unfortunate way when Leslie came home to find that Sam had sunk into a serious depression and had swallowed a large quantity of sleeping pills in an attempt to commit suicide. He was admitted to a hospital for psychiatric treatment, and this time he stayed with it. Since then, he has had no major recurrences of his disorder, and together Leslie and Sam have managed to build a real marriage and pay off some of their debts.

Bipolar illness (manic-depression) is classified as an *affective (mood) disorder*. The term refers to a mental problem in which the main disturbance is one of mood. The change in behavior and feeling may happen with no apparent cause, or be too extreme or long-lasting if a cause does exist.

Major affective (mood) disorders is the name given to mania (an elation bordering on psychosis or progressing to it), severe depression, or both. If a person's moods swing back and forth from extreme elation to deep depression, he is said to have a *bipolar disorder*. If his moods swing between normalcy and severe depression, or he stays depressed, he is said to have a *unipolar disorder*, or major depressive disorder. If he swings between full-blown, excited mania and normalcy, he is said to suffer from *manic episodes*.

Other affective disorders include *cyclothymic illness* (a chronic mood disturbance involving numerous periods of depression and a milder mania called hypomania, but not of enough severity and duration to be considered bipolar illness), and *dysthymic disorder* (a chronic mood disturbance involving either a depressed mood or loss of interest and pleasure in all usual activities and pastimes, but not of enough severity to be called major depressive illness).

Seasonal affective disorder (SAD) is a newly diagnosed condition in which depressive symptoms appear each year during seasons of decreasing daylight. People with this ailment crave carbohydrates, most severely during autumn and winter, when their depression is at its worst. These symptoms ease up in spring and summer. No one is sure why this happens, but one suggested treatment is tryptophan supplements, since a craving for carbohydrates could indicate low levels of the neurotransmitter serotonin. Many psychiatrists are treating SAD with a special fluorescent light apparatus called a SunBox, which mimics natural sunlight.

DEPRESSION

Of all the emotional problems discussed in this book, depression is the most common. Estimates vary, but many professionals say that 15-25 percent of the adult population suffers from serious depression at some time in their lives, and that 10 percent of the general population of America have clinical, severe depression and many do not know they need help.

Beverly was never a jolly person, but she managed to deal with the stresses and strains of life until she lost the beloved job she had held for 20 years. Not only could she not shake her extreme feelings of grief— even after many months—but her depression seemed to worsen with time. She began to pace around the house, wringing her hands and crying constantly. She couldn't get to sleep and had no desire to eat, which resulted in a 20-pound weight loss. Beverly began to believe she was a bad person and felt guilty about everything she had ever done. She even started to hear voices that told her she was totally worthless. When she finally sought help from her community mental health center, she was preoccupied with thoughts of suicide. Beverly was diagnosed as having major depression, and eventually recovered after professional treatment.

Not all depression requires treatment. The loss of a job, rejection by a lover, the death of a loved one—all of these can trigger *reactive depression*. It has an identifiable cause and the mood usually lifts with time. However, reactive depression can be serious if it lasts too long or is too severe. In these cases, the depressing incident may have triggered an underlying psychological problem.

Laurel, a 40-year-old teacher, was unnaturally attached to her mother. When the elderly woman died, Laurel stopped eating, speaking to people, or coming to work. She attempted to commit suicide. Her husband waited eight months, and when there was no improvement, he took her for treatment. She was placed on an antidepressant medication and saw a therapist once a week. After a few months, she began to improve dramatically and was soon back to normal.

Endogenous depression comes from within the person, and can have no cause. The symptoms vary widely from person to person (see list on opposite page):

- Angela enters her doctor's office and begins crying, telling him she is worthless and a burden to everyone she knows.
- John tells the doctor he is tired all the time and has started suffering from pains in his back, which shift their location from day to day.
- Larry sits staring at the floor and says he has no desire for food, sex, or life anymore.
- Rose feels fine mood-wise, but has lost her appetite, can't get to sleep,

and always feels tired. She moves and talks slowly.

• Marie says that nothing good will ever happen in her life, sleeps as much as 12 hours a day, eats constantly, and can become very anxious for no apparent reason.

We all experience highs and lows in our lives, but certain mood changes mark an affective mental disorder. These changes can be recognized by:

• intensity and duration
• problems with social relationships, either at home or work, or the loss of interest in hobbies or other forms of entertainment
• physical symptoms, such as sleep disturbances, appetite disturbances, reduced interest in sexual activity, and slowed motor movements
• misperception of reality, in which hallucinations, delusions, or confusion are present
• suicidal thoughts and behavior, or a loss of judgment that makes the person dangerous to himself or others.

SYMPTOMS OF DEPRESSION

sadness	sleeping problems
guilt	menstrual problems
hostility	loss of sexual interest
remorse	impotence
anger	weight loss
mood swings	fatigue or weakness
crying	unexplained pains in
slowed movements	various areas
agitated movements	poor self-image
withdrawal from life	indecisiveness
delusions	feelings of hopelessness,
hallucinations	helplessness, and
constipation	worthlessness
eating disorders	

Depressed patients may become hypochondriacal or manifest physical symptoms that have no biological cause (see Chapter Eight). They often do this as a cry for help, because if they are physically sick they can see a doctor without fear or embarrassment. Many physicians can spot this, and know when to refer their patients to a psychologist or psychiatrist for help.

Because all types of depression involve the risk of suicide, treatment must be quick and effective. Suicide is the tenth major cause of death in the United States and people with affective disorders have a 15 percent chance of killing themselves at some time in their lives. Among white males, aged 15 to 19, it is one of the major causes of death. Although more attempts are made by women in this country, men's attempts are more often successful. Throughout the world, the annual number of suicides is equal to the population of Edinburgh, Scotland, and the number who try to kill themselves equals the population of London or Los Angeles. In recent years, there has been a frightening rise among teenagers in both the appearance of depressive disorders and the incidence of suicide.

Studies indicate that there may be a genetic link in the development of unipolar depression. There is no conclusive evidence, but families with a history of clinical depression have a greater tendency to produce children suffering from the same disorder. On the biological front, several studies have suggested that a deficiency of the brain neurotransmitters serotonin or norepinephrine, or both, may be factors in depression. Some doctors feel that the onset of depression is often due to environmental stress, either combined with genetic tendencies and brain imbalances, or by itself.

Drugs Used to Treat Depressive Disorders

The treatment of depression has come a long way because much time and money has been spent researching affective disorders of all types. A combination of therapies are often used, including various types of psychotherapy, and if the depression is severe or suicidal tendencies are present, electroconvulsive treatments may be tried. In the early years of drug therapy, direct stimulants such as amphetamines were used, but these proved to be addictive and could cause anxiety or even psychotic symptoms. During the 1950s two better forms of drug treatment were introduced—the tricyclic antidepressants (TCAs) and the monoamine oxidase inhibitors (MAOIs). Both of them act by affecting the appropriate neurotransmitter levels in the brain. MAOIs are now more often used as a last resort when the TCAs don't work, because their many drug-drug and drug-nutrient interactions make them more dangerous. Recently, some new classes of antidepressants related chemically to the TCAs were released, and these appear to have far fewer side effects and may be less toxic in overdoses.

Many manic patients have depressive episodes. These are usually managed with lithium, unless the patient is in the severe depressive stage, when TCAs may be employed. The only danger with using antidepressants on bipolar patients is that the medication may trigger a manic episode in some patients. Antidepressants are almost never used when the mania is present.

Sedatives and antianxiety agents are prescribed when anxiety and tension accompany the depression. Antipsychotic drugs such as phenothiazines have proven helpful in treating very agitated depressed psychotic patients. For people with recurrent episodes of depression, maintenance therapy consists of antidepressants (where appropriate), plus supportive psychotherapy.

MANIA

What's wrong with feeling "up"? Many manic patients ask this question and resist treatment. But feeling good and being happy, or even elated, is not mania. This affective disorder is said to be present when elation is unreasonable, delusions are present, sleep is shunned, and various types of abnormal behavior appear (see list below).

Manic patients can go through several stages, not all of which are unpleasant. Hypomania may consist only of elation, increased energy, and bursts of creativity. In certain businesses, this is encouraged, because people in the hypomanic stage can be very creative and accomplish a great deal. Full-blown mania has the characteristics of psychosis—the person is often out of touch with reality, spends money madly, never goes to sleep, has hallucinations and delusions, and may be socially embarrassing, super-aggressive and even dangerously hostile.

In the most severe stage of mania, the patient may be delirious, with delusions of extreme grandeur ("I will save this planet now with my intergalactic mind rays"), disorientation, intense hostility, and an inability to complete a single thought.

SYMPTOMS OF MANIA

(Slight mania progresses to full psychotic mania,
then ends in deep depression.)

Slight mania
increased energy
increased capabilities
feelings of happiness

Mild Mania (Hypomania)
extreme optimism
decreased need for sleep
increased creativity
lack of judgment

talkativeness
impatience
obsession with sexual matters
aggressiveness
irritability
some loss of attention or ability to concentrate
no delusions
fairly normal speech

Full Mania (Hypermania)
spending money beyond financial capability
grandiose thoughts or belief in self-omnipotence
seductive sexual behavior, often to the point of indecency
extreme hostility, possibly leading to violent behavior
delusions of grandeur
loss of judgment
inability to concentrate
constant talkativeness and movement
arrogance
demanding, self-exalting behavior
making abusive or obscene statements
combativeness
nonsensical speech (sometimes)
shouting and throwing things
paranoid thoughts

Super-achievers and workaholic business executives may sometimes be functioning with a mild manic affective disorder—or bipolar illness— but their lifestyle or success stops them from seeking help. The problem with the manic stage is that judgment is impaired, and patients almost inevitably "crash" into bleak depression. Some put up with the down periods because they enjoy the highs so much.

Looking at the life of a gambler provides a good illustration of manic-depression. The compulsive gambler begins with a sense of elation and mastery over the game. His confidence and excitement build until he moves into manic "overdrive," where extravagance and loss of judgment begin to take over—making him an eventual loser. Whereas his hypomania works for him, his hypermania works against him, leading him into a "losing streak." After the eventual loss he may enter the depressed phase, where he can experience delusions of dire poverty— even if he has only lost a few hundred dollars. If a gambler is really suffering from an affective disorder, the gain or loss of money is not what triggers the emotions. In fact, his monetary status is an effect, rather than a cause, of his moods.

Genetic factors appear to play a significant part in bipolar, or manic-depressive, disorder. The results of two recent studies done on Amish families and five families in Jerusalem show that a genetic site can be linked to the disorder. The Amish study found a manic-depressive marker on chromosome 11; the Israeli research found a region on the X chromosome linked to the disease. Biochemically, mania has been theorized to result from a relative excess in the brain of the neurotransmitters dopamine, norepinephrine, or both.

Drugs Used to Treat Mania

The treatment of mania depends on its severity. People with hypomania are often helped as outpatients, whereas hospitalization is advised for those with an acute, full manic attack. The medication lithium shortens the periods of elation and helps prevent future attacks of either depression or mania when used as part of a maintenance program. Antipsychotic drugs, especially the phenothiazines and butyrophenones, are effective in controlling psychomotor agitation. Since it takes several days for lithium to become effective, lithium and an antipsychotic or an anti-anxiety agent, such as lorazepam, may be prescribed simultaneously for an acute manic attack. Some doctors favor using carbamazepine (Tegretol) as an alternative treatment for bipolar patients. Some are also using benzodiazepines (i.e., lorazepam or diazepam) instead of antipsychotics to control agitation during the acute manic phase. When the elation comes under control, the antipsychotic drug is gradually withdrawn. One of the many types of psychotherapy usually accompany drug treatment.

ARTISTS AND AFFECTIVE ILLNESS

What do Vincent Van Gogh, Handel, and Rossini have in common? It appears they all may have suffered from affective disorders. Handel wrote the entire score for the *Messiah* in just 6 weeks. Rossini wrote *The Barber of Seville* in just 13 days (an almost impossible feat unless the person was in manic overdrive). Van Gogh suffered from drastic mood changes, alternating between profound depression and extreme exuberance, ending with his suicide in July of 1890.

Are artists more prone to mood disorders? Many people used to think so, because their behavior often appears eccentric and their emotions are more evident. But modern therapists disagree. Although artists may be more likely to have problems with drugs, alcohol, suicidal thoughts, and mood changes than the rest of the population, they are creative in spite of any illnesses and not because of them. They also can be brilliant and have no emotional disorders. If they are more at risk, it is simply because they are often more emotionally vulnerable. They cannot and do not want to cut off incoming stimuli because it helps trigger the creative process.

Some mental-health professionals feel that creative artists who produce a lot in a short amount of time may be hypomanic, but not uncomfortable with their symptoms. Other creative people who do suffer from mania or hypomania are afraid of drug treatment, because they fear that if the illness goes, the art will go with it. By and large this has not been shown to be the case. In fact, many artists who have been placed on medication for treatment of disturbing symptoms show better judgment and produce more organized works of art. However, because stronger medication has reduced the creative drive in some people, the working artist may want to consider if he and others can tolerate his symptoms, or may decide to try medication and see if the benefits outweigh any losses.

THE CHEMISTRY OF MOOD

Mood changes can be the result of something that happens externally, internally, or from a brain biochemical balance. They may be a combination of all three. Biochemical mood swings can afflict women before the onset of their periods, or at certain times in the month, because of hormonal changes. Sometimes a trigger—such as stress at work—is needed to set off the disturbance, but in other cases, it happens without explanation.

A person or his loved ones must decide whether a mood disturbance is severe enough to demand treatment. If you are uncertain, it is best to consult with a therapist. You can ask yourself these questions:

• Has it lasted a long time?
• Does it recur?
• Are the symptoms uncomfortable, out of proportion to an event, or triggered mysteriously?
• Has the behavior, thoughts, physiology, or emotions changed in an unusual manner?

If the answer is "yes" to any of these questions, treatment is probably the answer. Sometimes drugs will not be prescribed, and short-term therapy is enough. On the other hand, the use of the appropriate medication can often erase the painful symptoms of a lifetime.

CHAPTER EIGHT

SOMATOFORM AND PSYCHOPHYSIOLOGIC DISORDERS: When the Mind Cripples the Body

Mrs. Carter considered herself a very fortunate woman, and rightly so. She had been married since the age of 19 to a man who doted on her, catering to her every need. He had grown very wealthy through hard work and fortunate investments, and so Mrs. Carter lived a life of luxury in a large apartment staffed by a maid and personal secretary. She enjoyed her days, shopping and lunching with friends and working for various charitable organizations. Although she could be difficult at times, prone to irritability and slight depressions, her husband knew how to soothe her—with affection, gifts, and trips to exotic places.

At the age of 64, Mr. Carter died unexpectedly of a heart attack. Although Mrs. Carter was well provided for, she sank into a severe depression. But after a year, it passed. She found herself a new apartment and a large circle of friends. She still grieved for her husband but appeared to be coping. However, a few months after settling into her new life, she began to complain of severe pains in her legs. Her daughter took her to the best specialists, but they could find nothing wrong. Eventually the pain became so severe she found it impossible to walk.

Again she underwent a battery of medical tests. The conclusion was the same: there was nothing wrong with her legs. More than one doctor suggested that the problem might be psychological. Finally, Mrs. Carter was taken to a psychotherapist. By this time, her depression had returned as well. As her paralysis worsened, she was eventually admitted to a clinic specializing in psychiatric disorders. After several years of intensive therapy and treatment with antidepressant medications, Mrs. Carter began to recover the use of her legs. Today she is leading a normal life, although she still finds it hard to believe that her severe pain and paralysis were caused by a mental disturbance.

Mrs. Carter's attitude is not unique. Many people cannot accept the fact that emotional problems can cause symptoms which mimic true physical illness. Others feel that the patients in question are exaggerating the pain or "faking it" to gain attention. But doctors know better. Victims of disorders that affect the body in some way feel the pain and are rarely in conscious control of their symptoms. Underlying emotional problems may trigger these physical symptoms, and until these conflicts are resolved, improvement is unlikely—no matter how much the patient wants to get better. In Mrs. Carter's case, her depression over her husband's death, coupled with her fear of having to run her life without him (and her reluctance to do so) resulted in physical paralysis—which again put her in a position where others had to take care of her, as she had been cared for in the past.

Sometimes severe depression alone is enough to trigger such symptoms. Patients who suffer from manic-depressive or depressive episodes can become frightened by their erratic behavior and do not want to ask for help, fearing institutionalization. Unconsciously, they then develop an illness. With specific physical symptoms, they can then go to a doctor. If the physician does not see the problem as masked depression, consequences as severe as suicide can result.

Disorders that affect the body are grouped under two broad categories—somatoform disorders (SD) and psychophysiologic disorders (PD). In the SD group, physical symptoms suggest a medical disorder, but organic evidence does not support this, and indications exist of an underlying emotional problem. These symptoms are not under the voluntary control of the patient. In PD cases, there *is* a physical condition that psychological factors have contributed to, either by starting it or exacerbating it. Such is the case with the eating disorder *anorexia nervosa*.

SOMATOFORM DISORDERS

The first type of SD is *somatization disorder*, which was also known as Briquet's syndrome or hysteria. It is characterized by recurrent and multiple physical complaints over several years, for which medical attention has been sought but has yielded no answers. This problem usually begins before the age of 30 and can last a lifetime. Patients often describe their physical complaints in a very dramatic or exaggerated way. Anxiety, depression, antisocial behavior, and problems with relationships and/or work are commonly found in these people. Their thoughts are often dominated by their symptoms, and they may lead lives as chaotic and complicated as their medical history. They go from doctor to doctor, refusing to believe there is no physical reason for their problems. Their preoccupations can lead to abuse of drugs such as painkillers.

Years ago, when I was in the hospital because of severe food poisoning, I shared a room with a very attractive housewife in her early forties. She was eager to tell me in graphic detail about her numerous physical problems, which included severe back pain and constant digestive upsets.

"Doctors are completely useless, all over the world," she said. "I've been to the best, and they can't find a thing. None of them take the right tests."

Not knowing any better, I believed her and felt sorry for this woman, who was obviously very sick and could find no adequate treatment. It seemed she had been suffering this way for over 15 years, could not work or enjoy herself, and felt doomed to a life of illness. Just before I left, I found her packing to leave the hospital.

"I guess I'll have to go somewhere else," she explained. "These doctors don't know anything either, so they're using the same old line— they say it's all in my mind. Imagine! They want me to see a psychiatrist, when my back is nearly paralyzed with pain, and I can't eat anything!"

Something in me started to see the light, but I did not answer at the time. The woman was hysterical, appeared to be suffering from too many diverse and extreme symptoms, and how was it that no doctor in the world could find anything wrong with her? Today it is clear to me that this woman was probably suffering from somatization disorder. I can only hope that her husband stopped indulging her complaints and did find adequate psychiatric care for her.

Conversion disorder (also known as hysterical neurosis of the conversion type) involves the loss of some type of physical function caused by emotional problems. The evidence of symptoms produces "secondary gain," as when men in combat develop paralysis of the arm and consequently do not have to fight. In fact, although this disorder is slightly more common in women, it is often found among men in a military setting. Many of these patients are so dramatic about their symptoms, and their secondary gain is so obvious, that people think they are consciously feigning or simulating the disease, when in actuality they have no conscious control over their symptoms.

The signs that mark conversion disorder can vary widely, but generally fall into two categories:

- Sensory problems, such as a diminished sense of pain, an absence of feeling, or a tingling sensation.
- Motor problems—such as convulsions, paralysis, muscular weakness, or aphonia (an inability to produce normal speech).

Doctors have come a long way toward understanding these disorders. Hippocrates believed they were caused by a wandering uterus. In the 17th century, hysteria was thought to be the result of demonic possession. Today we know that the main cause, or primary gain, is relief from anxiety. The secondary gain is the advantage that comes as a result of the illness—such as the ability to avoid doing or facing something unpleasant. A conversion disorder may also develop after a real illness if there is an underlying emotional problem. In this case, the hysteria prolongs or exaggerates the symptoms that originally resulted from the physical ailment.

Roger had just landed an excellent sales job, but his life was filled with problems. His marriage was on the rocks, and his young son was hyperactive. In addition, his new position was very demanding. Shortly before he was to give a presentation at an important sales conference, he became very ill, complaining of severe chest pain and difficulty in speaking. He thought his condition might be related to a viral infection or a heart problem, but the physical findings were negative. After he suffered twice more from the same type of "attacks" under similar conditions, he went to see a therapist and was diagnosed as having conversion symptoms.

Psychogenic pain disorder is another form of SD. The main symptom is intense pain with no physical cause. Something stressful in the environment may trigger it, and the patient can avoid facing the problem because of the debilitating symptom. In some cases, the pain may have a symbolic significance. Joseph was unnaturally attached to his father—he idolized him in every way. Several years after his father died from arteriosclerosis, Joseph began to suffer from angina pains, although doctors could find no cause for them. Joseph, whose business was failing, was simply trying to mimic his father, who had been enormously successful, by developing the same illness.

Hypochondriasis is the form of SD most of us are familiar with, although many people do not realize it is a recognized mental disorder. People with this problem unrealistically interpret physical signs or sensations as abnormal, leading to the fear or belief that they have a serious disease. A simple cough from a cold may be interpreted as a rare form of lung cancer; indigestion may be dubbed a minor heart attack. The hypochondriac is painfully aware of symptoms that other people ignore, such as slight fatigue or a headache.

On the other hand, people with this disorder often have trouble giving a precise description of their symptoms.

Somatization disorder and hypochondriasis are closely related. The main differences appear to be that hypochondriasis often starts after the age of 30, that exaggerated health complaints from a hypochondriac do not necessarily center around a particular set of symptoms, and that the hypochondriac fears having a disease rather than focusing on specific symptoms or physical disabilities.[1]

[1]Coleman, J.C., Butcher, J.N., and Carson, R.C. *Abnormal Psychology and Modern Life,* 7th edition, Scott Foresman & Co., 1984, p. 207.

Hypochondriacs are often preoccupied with digestive and excretory functions, and some even keep charts of their bowel movements. Many of them can give detailed information about diet, constipation, and related matters. These patients are frequently egocentric and overly concerned with themselves and their bodies. Others show obsessive-compulsive traits (see Chapter Six). Some experts believe that hypochondriacal adults are trying to gain attention and manipulate others through their constant complaints of illness. Again, one must remember that these people are convinced they are very sick, and they often need psychological help.

Treatment

For every type of somatoform disorder, supportive psychotherapy is a good place to start. Antianxiety agents are used for anxiety and antidepressants are used for depression, even though these drugs often have only temporary effects. However, they can relieve the symptoms of many types of somatoform disorders so therapy can be more successful.

PSYCHOPHYSIOLOGIC DISORDERS

Psychosomatic Gastrointestinal Reactions

There is a strong link between food, digestion, and emotions, so the mind-body connection is obvious with this common type of PD. The most frequent manifestation of this problem is a disease known as *anorexia nervosa*—the severe and prolonged refusal to eat, accompanied by extreme weight loss, disappearance of the menstrual period, impotence, disturbance of body image, and the fear of becoming obese. It is most often found in young girls and young women, although both sexes, at any age, can suffer from it. Its "sister" disease is *bulimia,* which is marked by periods of binge-eating followed by self-induced vomiting and/or the abuse of laxatives and diuretics (the latter behavior is also found in anorexia nervosa). Bulimics are often severely depressed as well, and while anorexics can die from starvation and malnutrition, bulimics are often prone to death from suicide.

Both of these eating disorders can be serious. The family and friends of such people should pay attention to any abnormal eating habits and seek help for the patient before it is too late. Treatment includes hospitalization, where some patients require constant observation in a locked psychiatric ward and tube-feeding. Behavioral therapy has also been successful in many cases. Some patients are treated with antidepressant drugs.

Recent studies at the National Institute of Mental Health are exploring the concept that people who have radically starved themselves below a certain weight experience a type of euphoria that reinforces their behavior. This feeling of well-being may be caused by increased secretions of endorphins (our natural opiates) in the brain. Researchers at Cambridge University in England are using the drug naltrexone (Trexan), which blocks the effects of opiates, with these patients. So far, the results have not been conclusive.

Obesity, in which a person's body weight exceeds by 20 percent or more what is normal according to standard height-weight tables, is often linked to depression or anxiety. Along with a revised diet, behavior modification, and an exercise program, appetite suppressants (mostly amphetamine or amphetamine-like compounds) may be prescribed for a short period of time. These drugs can be dangerous if taken over a prolonged period or in large quantities (causing addiction, insomnia, anxiety, and even psychotic-like symptoms). If severe depression or anxiety is present, the careful use of antianxiety or antidepressant drugs may be advised.

Psychosomatic Respiratory Disorders

Emotions such as hostility, anger, fear, or excitement can cause disruptions in respiration. *Hyperventilation syndrome* is one example, where the person suffers from repeated forced breaths, yawning, the sensation of a hunger for air, chest pains, muscle rigidity, tingling and numbness in the hands, feet, and face, lightheadedness, and sometimes the feeling of impending death due to suffocation. Some doctors feel that this is a rarely recognized form of anxiety disorder (see Chapter Six), and is often the result of disturbing dreams or nightmares. As in certain forms of panic disorder, the person awakens from a terrifying dream with fully developed symptoms. For these problems, psychotherapy combined with the use of antidepressants and antianxiety agents has proven very successful.

Asthma is an allergic disorder with labored breathing and wheezing due to a bronchial obstruction. The obstruction is caused by a spasm of the bronchial tubes, edema (collection of fluid in the lungs), and clumps of mucus that block off air passages. Emotional upsets can aggravate the condition. Tricyclic antidepressants may be used in combination with other drugs because they help open air passages, even though asthma often has no direct psychological cause.

Psychosomatic Musculoskeletal Disorders

This category includes a number of disorders, the most common one being tension headaches, which are often related to chronic anxiety. Antianxiety drugs such as benzodiazepines, which have muscle-relaxing properties, are very useful. Biofeedback, in which the patient is taught to consciously influence his own physiological processes, has also been used successfully.

Backaches and rheumatoid arthritis are other conditions that are exacerbated by stress, but patients with these disorders are usually treated medically in places such as pain centers. Individual treatment programs are designed to help patients cope with chronic pain.

Emotional Reactions to Physical Illness

A serious or prolonged ailment—such as diabetes, heart surgery, the amputation of a limb—can cause extreme anxiety or depression. The short-term use of antianxiety or antidepressant agents is advisable if these feelings become overwhelming.

If you or someone you are close to is suffering from physical symptoms, has sought medical attention from more than one doctor and no cause for the problem has been found, it may be advisable to seek psychological help. Medication coupled with therapy may be able to clear up the problem so a normal life, free from thoughts of pain or illness, can be regained.

CHAPTER NINE

Schizophrenic and Paranoid Disorders

During tax season, one friend said with a smile, "Every year I just know I'm going to be audited. I'm such a paranoid person you wouldn't believe it."

I have heard people remark about someone who became irritable for no apparent reason: "What do you expect? That man's schizophrenic, I tell you. You should work for him—you'd see."

The terms "schizophrenia" and "paranoia" are familiar to most of us, and are sometimes used casually to describe any type of abnormal behavior. In actuality, schizophrenic and paranoid disorders are serious illnesses. Although some of us may exhibit mild forms of the bizarre behavior symptomatic of these problems, most will never know what it is like to live inside the minds of such patients. Then again, neither illness is as hopeless as some may believe. It is possible, though not usual, for a person to suffer from one schizophrenic episode in his life and recover completely. Also, through the use of outpatient therapy and medication, people suffering from these disorders are often able to participate fully in everyday life and not have to spend the rest of their lives in an institution, as was previously the case.

SCHIZOPHRENIA

This term covers a large range of symptoms and can have many different causes and manifestations. Schizophrenic illnesses are usually of psychotic proportions, marked by disturbances in language and communication, thought, perception, mood, and behavior that last longer than six months. Reality may be distorted or misinterpreted in the patient's mind, and he or she may suffer from accompanying delusions or hallucinations. Behavior may be withdrawn, regressive, and bizarre. The symptoms can also not be attributed to any physical injury or illness.

No one knows the actual cause of schizophrenia, although it also appears to have some genetic link. Schizophrenic and paranoid behaviors, though belonging to two separate illnesses, often go hand in hand. The syndromes that are now classified as schizophrenic have been recognized for over 3000 years, although they have carried different labels at various times in history. Greek physicians in the fifth century B.C. called it "dementia" and distinguished it from "mania" and "melancholia."

A Swiss psychiatrist, Eugen Bleuler, first used the term "schizophrenia" (split mind) in 1911. He coined this word because he believed the illness was marked mainly by a disorganization of thought processes, a lack of coherence between thought and emotion, and an inward turning away from reality. The "splitting" was not meant to imply two or more personalities, as some believe, but rather a splitting within the intellect and between intellect and emotion. Cases of multiple personality are actually dissociative reactions, usually due to some form of stress, in which the patient manifests two or more complete systems of personality. This disorder is not classified as schizophrenia.

The Symptoms of Schizophrenia
There are so many symptoms associated with this disorder it would be impossible to list them all here. But some of the main ones include:

- Delusions, hallucinations, and the belief that the patient can control the thoughts and feelings of others, or be controlled in the same way. These delusions include "thought broadcasting"—the belief that one's thoughts are broadcast to the outside world; "thought insertion"—the belief that one's thoughts are not one's own but inserted into the mind; and "thought withdrawal"—the belief that thoughts have been removed from one's head.
- Speech where successive ideas appear unrelated or only slightly related to one another ("The apples were good today. My mother always said I'd become a fireman.").
- Moods showing flatness, blunting, or inappropriateness (laughing when a finger is cut).
- Fantasy and daydreaming that substitutes for reality ("I had tea with the Queen of England today and she was very interested in my ideas").
- Heightened ambivalence in which there is an exaggeration of coexisting opposite feelings or emotions for the same person, goal, thing, or situation ("I love my brother so much. I'd like to kill the lying creep").
- Disturbed motor movements, such as not moving at all, not reacting to anything, making too many movements, or making purposeless and bizarre gestures.

The particular combination of symptoms often indicates which of the many types of schizophrenia the patient has. It is also important to point out, without going into detail, that some types of behavior are similar to symptoms of the illness but do not qualify as full-blown schizophrenia. A *schizoaffective disorder*, for example, is really a depressive or manic syndrome that includes or develops with psychotic symptoms not usually seen in those disorders. These symptoms may be characteristic of schizophrenia, even though they are not the real illness.

A *schizophreniform disorder* is one in which the symptoms are identical to those of schizophrenia, but the duration of the problem is less than 6 months but more than 2 weeks. A *schizotypal personality* has many irregularities such as egocentricity, avoidance of others, and eccentricity of speech, thought, and perception, but none of these are severe enough to meet the criteria for schizophrenia.

The Schizophrenic Patient

Jerry, a 19-year-old college student, was brought to the hospital by the police after having knocked on the door of a stranger's house at three in the morning, telling the woman who answered it that the Lord had sent him to use her special bathroom. Two years earlier, he had suffered a "nervous breakdown," as his parents called it, was hospitalized for six months and released, although his behavior continued to be withdrawn and sometimes bizarre.

Three days before Jerry was brought to the hospital, he had spent the night on his knees in front of the family fireplace, chanting and praying. The next day he started off for school, but in response to "voices," prayed in various churches around the neighborhood instead. He tried to attend school again the following morning, but became confused and had to come home, claiming that one of the girls in his classes was "blocking" his thoughts and mixing him up. He could not sleep again, was irritable and restless, and finally started to wander the streets in the clothes he had been wearing steadily for the last three days, ending up at the stranger's house.

Upon admission to the hospital, it was obvious that Jerry was seriously disturbed. He was preoccupied with ideas about morality and the nature of "true religion," and said that God constantly communicated with him through radio and television broadcasts. He called the doctors "his disciples," and warned them against "satanic forces." His mood was euphoric, he talked rapidly and often incoherently, flipping from one thought to the next with no connection. He also could not sit still, but kept walking around or assuming different odd postures for a few minutes at a time. At one point, he calmly exposed himself to a nurse.

Jerry became hostile and abusive at times, and once tried to injure himself by repeatedly slamming his head against a wall. After a three-month stay in the hospital, where he received therapy, electroconvulsive treatments, and antipsychotic medications, his behavior improved to some degree. He was committed to a state hospital to receive further care.

Schizophrenia occurs in less than one percent of the population. It may actually be several different disorders classed into one. At this point, there is little doubt in the medical community that biological factors play a role in development of the disease. Some experts strongly feel there is a genetic predisposition in these patients, although others point out that subsequent factors, such as stress in the environment, are needed to set it off. Studies do indicate that children of schizophrenic parents are more likely to develop the disorder than children from normal households.

In 1978, Dr. E. Kringlen showed that in families where both parents became schizophrenic at some point in their adult lives, 20 percent of the children developed clinical schizophrenia.

Researchers in the 1970s thought schizophrenia might be caused by the secretion of a chemical in the brain that resembled LSD or mescaline, a sort of endogenous hallucinogen. That theory is no longer considered a very likely explanation, nor is a more recent one—that schizophrenia is caused by an excess of the neurotransmitter dopamine in the brain. There is now interest in the possibility that the brain's natural opiates, endorphins and enkephalins, may be implicated in the development of disease. However, because nothing is conclusive, the biological riddle of schizophrenia remains unsolved at this time.

Environmental factors that may contribute to schizophrenia include broken homes, an upbringing in an impoverished area, and/or child abuse. Also, a child reared in a mentally unstable environment, in which the parents have schizophrenia or other psychotic disorders, is often at risk for development of the disease.

Treatment of Schizophrenia

Schizophrenia was once considered a progressive illness with a poor or hopeless prognosis. Today doctors recognize that there are episodic forms of the disease, and a patient can remain free of any symptoms for an extended period of time. Treatment of the disorder involves many types of therapy, both in and out of the hospital, and sometimes in halfway houses.

As far as drug therapy goes, it is most successful when used in combination with other therapeutic methods. It is difficult to get these patients to stick to their drug regimen after they are discharged from a hospital, and many patients suffer a relapse of symptoms when the drugs are withdrawn. The medications of choice for this illness are the antipsychotic agents, in many cases a phenothiazine. Sometimes intramuscular injections of a long-acting type of phenothiazine, such as Prolixin (fluphenazine), or a butyrophenone, such as haloperidol, are used.

PARANOIA

As mentioned, many schizophrenics also suffer from symptoms of paranoid illness. People with these disorders often project their own fears or shortcomings onto other people or events. They are overalert, highly suspicious, and suffer from delusions and a distorted view of reality. They feel singled out and taken advantage of, mistreated, plotted against, ignored, spied on, or otherwise abused by their "enemies."

The term paranoia literally means thinking *beside* oneself. Looking back in history, we find it was used synonymously with the term "insanity." Paranoid patients often show superior intellect and have many suppressed feelings, such as ones of extreme inferiority. Some people suggest there is a genetic factor involved in the development of the disease, but studies have not yet been conclusive in this area.

The Paranoid Patient

David, a 50-year-old single man, was brought to the hospital by his elderly parents. He repeatedly protested that he was not sick. About a year before, David had seen a physician because of back pains. He now said the doctor had given him strange injections designed to make him feel worse. He told his therapists that his father was in league with government officials in an attempt to try and get "his property" away from him. (He did not own property.) He also suspected his mother of telling department stores not to sell him anything and garages not to fix his car properly. David refused to work at an outside job, because he believed "spies" sent to find and capture him could more easily pinpoint his location at an office, where he would be surrounded by "double agents." He accused his neighbors of putting substances in the water to destroy the trees and grass. He had written many letters to politicians complaining of the latter practice, and had even sent soil and water samples to the U.S. Department of Agriculture. David was diagnosed as suffering from paranoia.

The Delusions of Paranoia

Paranoid people are filled with delusions about reality. These can take many forms:

• Erotic delusions. These can concern infidelity, sexual exploitation, change of sex, or the idea of being loved by some stranger—often a famous person who cannot publicly admit to the relationship.
• Jealous delusions. Here the jealousy is more persistent and profound than a normal person's would be, or there may be nothing to support the feeling at all.
• Grandiose delusions, such as having great power, fame, intellect, influence, or wealth.
• Persecutory delusions, which often accompany the grandiose ones. In this case, the paranoid patient feels he is being spied on, followed, slandered, or that his mind is being controlled or influenced by others. He may even believe a great conspiracy has been organized for his destruction.

Treatment of Paranoid Disorders

Various antipsychotic drugs, especially the phenothiazines, can be of some help in calming delusions and assisting the patient to again adapt to reality. Paranoid people rarely have to stay in mental hospitals, although therapy in these cases can become a tricky process. The doctor can become part of the patient's delusionary structures, so only those practitioners experienced in treating this disorder usually attempt the task.

While schizophrenic and paranoid disorders are extremely serious, neither implies a hopeless situation. Although antipsychotic drugs cannot cure the condition (any more than they can "cure" many other disorders), they may alleviate the symptoms and help these patients lead normal lives. However, as pointed out in the beginning of this book, therapy must also accompany medication. Patients should be monitored so that they know to take their drugs at specific times, and the seriously ill would probably be better served in a hospital environment.

CHAPTER TEN

FINDING THE RIGHT DOCTOR:
The Road to Healing

Some of the people reading this book are already under treatment for emotional problems. Others are being treated without the use of drugs and want to explore this road. Still others have recently been prescribed a medication and are not sure how it works and what they should know about its safety.

But there is another group of readers—those who have never tried psychological treatment, or who have in the past and were not pleased with the results. These people may be experiencing uncomfortable symptoms and are not sure what to do about them—or are simply frightened or ashamed.

So it is best to set the record straight. Not all people who are suffering from uncomfortable symptoms need professional help. Reactive depression, for instance, where an understandably upsetting event (the death of a spouse, the loss of a job) touches off a bad case of the "blues," may be quite normal and disappear in time. Anxiety triggered by a child's illness or a natural disaster (such as a fire or flood) may also be completely expected and short-lived. Only when these conditions last for a long period of time (over six months), are debilitating, or include thoughts of suicide, should treatment be sought. If the symptoms are bearable and do not interrupt a person's social life or work, and if they seem to be improving with time, the person may be able to resolve the problem by himself.

Another point that should be made is that seeking psychological help when it is needed is no longer (nor ever should have been) a reason for fear or embarrassment. Some doctors state that one in three people in the U.S. has an emotional problem that might require therapy. This emphasizes that one should not be ashamed of such symptoms. Not every problem can be dealt with by the individual himself. Often an outside, objective and professional counselor is the best medicine. If your health insurance does not cover such treatment, there are many clinics, group situations, and practices involving sliding scale payments based on your income that any doctor or hospital will gladly tell you about. So money should not be a deterrent either.

As we have pointed out, the field has grown so much that therapy need not involve years of time and significant amounts of money. We also now understand enough about the brain to say that mental illness should be regarded in the same way as physical illness—one is often a biological imbalance in the mind, the other in the body. So if you are suffering from symptoms that you wish to be rid of, or even if you simply want to understand more about yourself and become as effective as possible in your life, therapy is the best answer.

It is important not to lie to yourself about your own problems or those you see in the ones you love. The consequences of this can be serious, even fatal. Too many people justify symptoms and live with emotional pain, simply because they're afraid they might be "going crazy." Very few are. Most people just have a simple problem that can be corrected with the right therapy and medication.

The symptoms described in this section of the book are very general. Even though you may be exhibiting some of them, don't jump to the conclusion that you have the disorder described. Only a qualified professional can decide that. But if you are suffering from a moderate or serious disorder, that is a good reason to seek proper advice and treatment.

A simple analogy should make this clear. If you broke your arm, would you go home and sit in pain? Well, the same is true for mental health. Today our society has the expertise, the facilities, the medication to heal that pain. Use them. The stresses and strains of modern society are causing more people to seek help. And now, more than ever, problems can be solved.

If you are suffering from minor depression or anxiety, the first thing you may want to do is visit your local library or bookstore and look at some self-help books dealing with the topic. Many offer practical advice and exercises that may work for you. Eating a sound diet and starting a regular exercise program can also improve the condition, along with finding a hobby, learning a new skill, taking courses at school just for the fun of it, and generally getting out more and having a good time. If these simple techniques work, add them to your life—even if you still choose to see a therapist. But none of these simple solutions will solve a deep-rooted, serious problem. Recurrent symptoms must be treated professionally.

How do you find the right analyst, or change doctors if the current one doesn't seem to be helping? First, call the American Medical Association (AMA), American Psychiatric Association (APA), or other local mental-health organizations. They have brochures and names to offer and can be most helpful. Talk to friends who are undergoing analysis to see if they have recommendations. Best of all, consult your local nurse or family doctor who knows your history. They encounter depressed or troubled people in their day-to-day practice and usually have a list of psychiatrists to recommend. You may also want to visit a major medical center in your area—many have established psychiatric clinics, and much of the most up-to-date research is conducted in such facilities.

How do you find the most up-to-date doctors, well-versed in using the medications mentioned here? You should know that only psychiatrists can prescribe medications (psychologists are not M.D.'s), but many times psychologists work with psychiatrists who prescribe medications for the psychologists' patients. Although the words "doctor" and "psychiatrist" have been used most often in this book, it is simply because the emphasis is on drug therapy and only medical doctors can prescribe drugs. It is not meant in any way to indicate that psychologists or psychiatric social workers cannot treat a patient just as well. In cases where no medication is needed, a medical doctor may not even be brought into the picture.

People are often limited by their impression of doctors as "god figures." Patients are reluctant to ask enough questions or change doctors if they are unsatisfied with the treatment. This should by no means be the case. Once you get a name, make an appointment for a consultation, and see if you and the doctor "hit it off." One must look at it that way because successful therapy is often hinged upon a good and trusting relationship between doctor and patient. Of course, the therapist may sometimes say things that don't please you—it is often those items that we refuse to admit about ourselves that are causing the problem. But the proof comes with time. If you are showing no improvement, then seek a consultation visit with another doctor and see what he or she has to say. Usually, in these visits (especially in the case of minor problems), the patient will describe his or her symptoms and the doctor will roughly indicate the type of treatment he will use. This is where you can find out whether medications will or will not be used. If they are not mentioned, ask why. There may be a good reason, such as a contraindication in your medical history. Of course, a therapist cannot explain everything he or she is doing in treatment, because in some cases this would defeat the process of trying to make you see things you may never have admitted to yourself.

There are few bad doctors—but some suit a certain type of patient or problem better than others. Women may or may not prefer to see a woman physician, and the same applies to men. But again, this is not a rule. The doctor you can communicate with, who helps you, is the right one.

In the case of more serious problems, friends or families of patients may have to take the initiative. Very disturbed people often think of themselves as normal, because they have little touch with reality. But again, one must not let the patient be railroaded into a hospital or a treatment program without careful examination and a second opinion. Remember, in these cases, a whole life may be at stake.

Your Relationship with Your Doctor

If you are in therapy and medication has not been prescribed, suggest to your doctor the possibility of using it as an adjunct to therapy. Ask about any potential side effects or cautions. Make sure you are clear about what drugs, foods, or drinks should not be taken along with the medicine.

Once you are taking medication, you must continue therapy and check in with your doctor constantly, especially if you suspect you are having some adverse reactions. Take the medication at the times specified by your doctor. Forgetting to take a pill three times and then taking all of the missed pills at once can result in a toxic overdose. With some psychoactive medications, blood levels must be constantly checked in the first few weeks or months of treatment.

Remember, therapy will not be successful unless you are totally honest with your doctor. Don't pretend to feel better when you don't because you think it will please the therapist. He or she will be most satisfied when your health is restored.

PART TWO

DRUGS USED
TO TREAT ILLNESS

INTRODUCTION:
The Uses of Psychoactive Drugs

The following section lists the primary drugs used in the treatment of various psychological disorders. Not all drugs are covered here—only those in popular use for emotional problems of varying degrees, and which are available in this country.

These drugs fall into broad chemical groups (drug "families") made up of individual drugs that have very similar chemical makeup and action. There is a general entry for each group, with specific drugs and varying side effects for each drug listed within the entries. Drugs are mentioned by their generic (chemical compound) names first, accompanied by their brand names in parentheses. Ask your doctor if your drug is available in generic form, because these can be as effective and are usually less expensive than the brand-name version.

Side effects—as well as beneficial results—will vary from person to person. You may have to try a few drugs in a category to find one that alleviates your symptoms with the fewest or no adverse effects. Always keep your doctor informed of any reactions (some go away after a few days of use or with a decreased dosage).

Do not obtain these drugs from anyone other than a physician who is knowledgeable about their use—preferably a specialist in the psychological field. Never buy them illegally, as you cannot be sure of what you are buying. Further, abuse or overdose can be very dangerous. Take them in the prescribed doses at the recommended times. In most cases, they are meant to be used as an adjunct to professional therapy. With some medications, blood levels must be closely monitored by your doctor.

Check all drug-drug and drug-nutrient interactions. In the case of MAO inhibitors (antidepressant category), eating certain foods while taking them can cause a severe elevation in blood pressure. When you are taking a psychoactive drug, always inform a new doctor or a hospital admitting staff of that fact, either by bringing the bottle with you or knowing the name and dose level of the drug you are taking. One young woman almost died because her family failed to inform doctors in the emergency room where she was admitted after a car accident that she was taking MAO inhibitors. Not knowing this fact, the physicians administered another medication that can cause death when combined with an MAO inhibitor.

Each drug entry which follows is set up in the following way:

GENERIC NAMES

These are the chemical names of the drugs.

BRAND NAMES

These are brand names that are currently available and in popular use in the U.S. Many medications are sold under only one brand name.

USES

This lists medical conditions that are usually treated with the drug. Sometimes a physician may decide to use the drug for another reason because of individual body chemistry and/or problems.

ACTION

This describes how the drug is thought to work in the body to bring about beneficial effects. In some cases, this is not yet thoroughly known or proven.

USUAL DOSAGE

This is the recommended dose range for the drug. Because individuals may require different amounts of these drugs for effectiveness or safety, the actual dosage level is always determined by the doctor.

CONTRAINDICATIONS

These are conditions, such as pregnancy or heart disease, which make the use of certain drugs extremely dangerous or possibly fatal. However, sometimes in emergencies a physician may decide to administer the drug, albeit with utmost caution. In some cases, conditions where the safety of the drug has not been established are included in this category.

CAUTION

There are things to watch out for while taking specific drugs (such as driving a car because of heavy sedative effects), and conditions that demand close supervision while certain drugs are being used (such as kidney or liver problems).

SIDE EFFECTS

In this category, those side effects most common to the whole group of drugs are listed in the general entry (i.e., constipation in MAO inhibitors); adverse effects most often seen with the use of specific drugs are also included.

DRUG-DRUG INTERACTIONS

This details what and how other drugs affect the drug's action, and vice versa. Some drugs are dangerous in combination with others, some drugs combine to make both stronger, and others combine to make one stronger and the other weaker.

DRUG-NUTRIENT INTERACTIONS

This explains how the drug relates to food and beverages and lists which substances not to consume while using it. It also mentions if weight is affected in any way.

In most cases, drugs don't cure emotional/psychological disorders— they alleviate the symptoms. Only time, the willingness to change, the desire to get better, and professional help can bring about a total cure.

New drugs are being discovered all the time. Some have fewer side effects, take a shorter time to work, or are less likely to cause psychological or physiological dependency. Doctors in this field are very aware of new discoveries and medications, and are usually quite willing to answer any questions you may have. If you have one, by all means, ask.

GENERAL GUIDELINES FOR USING PSYCHOACTIVE MEDICATIONS

1. Take only the dose recommended by your doctor.
2. Do not combine these drugs with alcohol or other CNS depressants such as barbiturates unless approved by your doctor; combine them only with drugs prescribed by the doctor.
3. Do not obtain these drugs illegally; have them prescribed by a doctor who is well acquainted with their use.
4. Do not stop taking them abruptly because you feel better unless instructed to do so by your doctor. In most cases these drugs must be

gradually withdrawn in order to avoid adverse effects.

5. Inform your doctor of any side effects you might be experiencing.

6. Recognize that in many cases these drugs only relieve symptoms and must be accompanied by professional therapy and possibly a change in life attitudes and behavior.

7. Do not let yourself become either physically or psychologically dependent on these medications—tell your doctor if you feel you are having this type of problem.

8. Recognize that many of these drugs have sedative effects and so driving a car or operating machinery can be hazardous.

9. In cases of overdose, rush the patient to the hospital immediately.

CHAPTER ELEVEN

Antidepressants

Antidepressant agents certainly represent the tremendous break-throughs in treatment resulting from the use of current psychoactive drugs. Previous to their discovery and use, people with major bouts of depression were treated with electroconvulsive therapy (ECT), pro-longed hospitalization, or sedation—which often made the problem worse. People with mild depressive illness were treated with analysis. Although ECT is still used in combination with these drugs when the problem is severe—and therapy should always go hand-in-hand with their use—people no longer have to suffer from the crippling symptoms of this disorder while the full treatment is going on. Since depression is one of the most common psychiatric problems, these drugs are es-pecially important to all of us.

There are two major types of antidepressants now in use—the tricy-clics and the monoamine oxidase inhibitors (TCAs and MAOIs, respec-tively). The MAOIs are now often used as a last resort, since their numerous drug-nutrient and drug-drug interactions make them a great-er health risk. To be completely accurate, antidepressant agents are classed into four groups—therapeutic stimulants, TCAs, MAOIs, and tetracyclics and the new antidepressants—but the latter two are merely chemical alterations in similar compounds to the TCAs.

Stimulants like amphetamines are not really used anymore in treating depression, since they can cause insomnia, addiction, anorexia, severe anxiety, and even psychotic symptoms if taken in large doses for a long period of time. The only stimulants which are still used in cases of mild depression, and which we have included here in the last entries, are methylphenidate HCL (Ritalin) and pemoline (Cylert), although they are mainly employed in the treatment of hyperactivity in children.

The first TCA was discovered in 1940 and called imipramine, but it was not until 1958 that the compound was found to help depressed patients. In the case of the MAOIs, the antituberculosis drugs called isoniazid and iproniazid were found to have mood-elevating effects in 1951. In 1952, doctors discovered that iproniazid inhibited the action of the enzyme monoamine oxidase. From there, researchers concluded that it could be used in psychiatric treatment, since a low level of amine neurotransmitters in the brain might be responsible for depression, and monoamine oxidase breaks these transmitters down. By inhibiting its action, the levels could be raised and the symptoms of depression alleviated.

While antidepressant medications are relatively safe and can be used in conjunction with therapy for an extended period of time, there are many common side effects, and certain people who should not use them. Also, anyone taking these drugs should be aware of their drug-drug and drug-nutrient interactions (particularly in the case of the MAOIs).

MONOAMINE OXIDASE INHIBITORS (MAOIs)

GENERIC AND BRAND NAMES

isocarboxazid *(Marplan)*
phenelzine sulfate *(Nardil)*
tranylcypromine sulfate *(Parnate)*

USES

These drugs are mostly used in the treatment of certain types of depression, certain phobic-anxiety states, anxiety with hypochondriacal or hysterical features, and can be prescribed for bulimia, post-traumatic reactions, obsessive-compulsive disorders, and narcolepsy. People who have not shown any improvement on other types of antidepressants are often helped by these drugs. However, MAOIs are usually not the first drugs selected for treatment, because their drug-drug and drug-nutrient interactions can have serious consequences. In addition, as little as six to ten times the normal daily dose can be highly toxic, even lethal. The beneficial effects of these drugs may not be apparent for two weeks or more, and it can require an additional one to two weeks before they reach their maximum effectiveness.

ACTION

These drugs block the breakdown of amine neurotransmitters in the brain, leading to increases in the level of norepinephrine, serotonin, and dopamine.

USUAL DOSAGE

If the MAOI is too stimulating, it should not be given after 5 p.m.

isocarboxazid—Initially, up to 30mg daily in single or divided doses; maintenance dose can be 10-50mg daily.

phenelzine sulfate—15mg three times a day, increased if necessary to four times a day after two weeks, then reduced gradually to the lowest possible maintenance dose (as little as 15-60mg every day or every other day). Some patients do not respond until treatment with 60-90mg per day has been continued for at least four weeks.

tranylcypromine sulfate—Initial dose is 20mg a day—10mg in the morning and 10mg in the afternoon (usually no later than 3 p.m.)—for two weeks. If no improvement is seen, dosage can be increased to 30-60mg a day. This treatment is usually continued for one week; if there is still no improvement, the drug is discontinued. Maintenance dose can be reduced to 10-20mg daily.

CONTRAINDICATIONS
Not recommended for patients with heart disease, a history of strokes, liver disease, epilepsy, and hyperthyroidism, as well as most elderly patients, debilitated patients, and children under 12 years of age.

CAUTION
These drugs may affect mental concentration and the ability to drive a car or operate machinery. Avoid abrupt discontinuation. This treatment can cause hypomania (a milder form of mania) in patients with disorders in which hyperactive symptoms exist, but are obscured by depression. In these cases, hypomania usually appears after the depression subsides. If agitation is present, the drugs may increase it. Hypomania and agitation sometimes appear with high doses of these drugs or after prolonged use. They may also cause psychotic episodes in schizophrenic patients. In manic-depressives, a swing from the depressive to the manic stage may be seen. It is not known whether or not these drugs may be used with safety in pregnant or lactating women.

A waiting period of about two weeks is required to change from treatment with tricyclic antidepressants (TCAs) to MAOIs. This is to avoid the rare but serious reactions (such as excitability, cardiovascular changes and nausea) that can be caused by taking both drugs at the same time. Also, some people are sensitive to these drugs and should not use them. This sensitivity will manifest itself with side effects almost immediately, even with low doses. Therefore, all side effects should be reported to the physician.

SIDE EFFECTS

Antidepressant medications may have the same anticholinergic (chemical action that blocks the effect of the neurotransmitter acetylcholine) side effects invoked by antipsychotic drugs—dry mouth, sweating, blurred vision, and constipation. (However, MAOIs rarely cause these effects.) Central nervous system effects include drowsiness, agitation, and a fine tremor. These drugs may, in rare cases, cause hallucinations and delusions in patients who appear depressed but are latently psychotic, and can cause impotence or sexual frigidity, and weight gain.

isocarboxazid—Side effects tend to be mild to moderate in severity and often subside as treatment continues or when the dosage is reduced. They include: dizziness and low blood pressure (hypotension) upon standing, agitation, headache, tremor, constipation, dry mouth, blurred vision, difficulty in urinating, liver damage, and skin rash.

phenelzine sulfate—Same general side effects appear, but also swelling in the legs and ankles (edema) are rarely seen.

tranylcypromine sulfate—Insomnia, dizziness, muscular weakness, dry mouth, low blood pressure. Hypertensive crisis (very high blood pressure), with throbbing headache requiring cessation of treatment, occurs more frequently with this drug than with the other MAOIs, whereas liver damage occurs less frequently.

DRUG-DRUG INTERACTIONS

MAOIs do not combine well with many drugs, including stimulants such as amphetamines, fenfluramine, levodopa, caffeine, and over-the-counter drugs containing stimulants (cold medications, nasal decongestants, hay-fever medications, sinus medications, asthma inhalants, appetite suppressants, weight-reducing preparations, and "pep" pills). Use with these types of drugs can lead to very high blood pressure, the first symptom of which is usually a throbbing headache. Tricyclic and related antidepressants should not be given until 14 days after treatment with MAOIs has been stopped. The effects of antidiabetic drugs are increased.

DRUG-NUTRIENT INTERACTIONS

MAOIs should be taken with meals or milk, because these drugs sometimes cause gastrointestinal distress.

Knowledge of the drug-nutrient interactions these drugs have is extremely important. Toxic reactions to cheese and other foods containing amines, such as tyramine, dopamine, histamine or tyrosine, are likely to occur. The attacks are marked by transient but often critically high blood pressure, headaches, nausea, vomiting, and palpitations. A stroke or even death can be caused by this reaction. The severity of the attacks has been linked to the level of tyramine in particular foods. The ingested tyramine is usually converted in the liver to an inactive form through the action of monoamine oxidase (MAO). Because MAOIs leave tyramine in its active form by blocking the action of MAO, it remains in the blood where it can raise the blood pressure to dangerous levels. Reactions usually occur within a half hour of consuming the offending food or drink.

Foods containing dopa or dopamine have similar effects. Other antidepressant drugs, such as amphetamines, also act as MAOIs, and when combined with tyramine and dopamine-containing foods can cause very serious or even lethal side effects. Similar problems have been observed with caffeine in animal experiments.

Tyramine is found in the greatest amounts in high-protein foods that have undergone some decomposition, such as aged cheese (especially Swiss, cheddar, brie, camembert, gruyere, and blue cheese.) It is also found in raisins, plums, avocados, chicken and beef livers, bananas, eggplant, sauerkraut, yogurt, sour cream, alcoholic beverages (especially sherry, beer, and Chianti wine), salami, meat tenderizers, coffee, pepperoni, frankfurters, pickled herring, fava or broad beans, cola, chocolate, canned figs, pineapples, yeast and soy sauce. Raisins and avocados also contain dopamine. Anyone taking MAOIs should avoid all these foods, but some (i.e., yogurt, sour cream, avocado, chocolate, caffeine-containing beverages, clear spirits, white wine, and soy sauce) may be taken in moderation.

These drugs can increase appetite and lead to weight gain.

WARNING

If you or someone you know is taking MAOIs and has an extreme reaction, go to the hospital emergency room. It is not wise to simply lie down and hope the reaction will pass, because it could be the start of a hypertensive crisis and must be treated professionally. In all cases, report any unusual side effects to your doctor.

TRICYCLIC ANTIDEPRESSANTS (TCAs)

(This category includes the tetracyclics and newer antidepressants, which are simply chemical modifications of similar compounds, and in some cases have fewer side effects.)

GENERIC AND BRAND NAMES

Tricyclic Antidepressants
amitriptyline hydrochloride *(Elavil, Endep)*
desipramine hydrochloride *(Norpramin, Pertofrane)*
doxepin hydrochloride *(Adapin, Sinequan)*
imipramine hydrochloride *(Janimine, SK-Pramine, Tofranil)*
imipramine pamoate *(Tofranil-PM)*
nortriptyline hydrochloride *(Pamelor, Aventyl)*
protriptyline hydrochloride *(Vivactil)*

Newer Antidepressants
maprotiline hydrochloride *(Ludiomil)*
amoxapine *(Asendin)*
trazodone hydrochloride *(Desyrel)*
trimipramine maleate *(Surmontil)*

USES
These drugs are the treatment of choice for depression and are said to produce an overall improvement rate of 70 percent. They are most effective for moderate to severe depression associated with psychological and psychomotor changes such as loss of appetite and sleep disturbances (improvement in sleeping habits is usually the first benefit). Treatment with TCAs for two to three weeks may be necessary before any positive changes are seen, and patients should be checked frequently in the early weeks of treatment for any suicidal tendencies. Newer antidepressants take effect more quickly. Remission of symptoms usually occurs three months to one year after therapy begins, but each patient is unique. To prevent relapse, some people then benefit from several months of treatment, with 50 percent of the therapeutic dose found to be effective.

Although anxiety may be the most prominent symptom in depressive illness, antipsychotic and antianxiety drugs are used with caution, as they can mask the underlying depression. However, they may be used to treat agitated depression, and in the early stages of treatment it is often appropriate to add a sedative to correct sleeping problems and an antianxiety drug when agitation is severe.

The symptoms most likely to respond to treatment with these drugs include:

- appetite and sleep disturbances
- decreased energy
- decreased sexual function and/or interest
- psychomotor agitation or retardation

- diurnal mood variations (where the depression is worse in the morning)

The symptoms least likely to respond are:

- a low sense of self-esteem
- feelings of hopelessness or helplessness
- demoralization

There is no need for this type of treatment when the depression is reactive and justified (clearly related to circumstances or incidences in one's environment). These drugs are sometimes used for manic depression and schizoaffective disorders, but lithium is usually the drug of choice for long-term management of chronic manic-depression, whereas these antidepressants are employed for acute depressive attacks. However, they may trigger a manic episode and so must be used with caution in this situation.

From 10-20 percent of all patients do not respond to these drugs, in which case an MAOI may be prescribed; a two-week interval must be allowed before changing from one to the other, because combining both medications is extremely hazardous.

Additional information (where appropriate):

amitriptyline—Depression where anxiety is also present, because it has additional sedative properties.

doxepin hydrochloride—Anxiety and depression associated with alcoholism, depression where anxiety is present, and major depressive disorders including manic-depression (bipolar illness).

protriptyline hydrochloride—Useful for withdrawn patients lacking in energy and apathetic; it has a stimulating action and produces the least amount of sedation.

maprotiline hydrochloride—Depression with anxiety or depressive neurosis (dysthymic disorder).

amoxapine—Depression with anxiety.

trazodone hydrochloride—Depression with anxiety, but a good choice if some sedation is required early in treatment.

trimipramine maleate—Depressive illness especially when associated with anxiety and insomnia, because of its sedative effects.

One must again realize, however, that certain drugs work better on certain people, and that there is no hard-and-fast rule concerning which drug will be most effective for a specific person. Only a physician can make the decision.

ACTION

While no one yet understands fully how these drugs alleviate the symptoms of depression, one way in which they appear to work is by increasing the levels of norepinephrine and serotonin in the brain. They block retrieval of these neurotransmitters by the neurons (nerve cells), holding them instead in the synapses between the nerve cells. Although it has not yet been conclusively proven, depression is believed to be related in part to a low level of these biogenic amine neurotransmitters in the central nervous system.

USUAL DOSAGE

amitriptyline hydrochloride—In adults, initial dose is 50-75mg in divided portions, or as a single dose at bedtime. This can be increased gradually to a maximum dose of 150-300mg a day. Taking the medication at night helps promote sleep and avoids daytime drowsiness. Maintenance dose is 50-100mg a day. In the elderly and adolescents, a lower dose of 25-50mg in divided doses or a single dose at bedtime should be used.

desipramine hydrochloride—In adults, 75mg is taken daily in divided doses or as a single dose at bedtime, gradually increased if necessary to 200-300mg a day. Maintenance dose is usually the lowest dose that will preserve remission. In the elderly and adolescents, 25mg can be raised to 150mg if needed.

doxepin hydrochloride—For mild to moderate anxiety and/or depression, an initial dose of 10-25mg is given three times a day; this may be increased gradually to 75-150mg daily. For more severe cases, the dose may be 150-300mg given in divided doses. Up to 100mg can be given as a single dose at bedtime.

imipramine hydrochloride—Hospitalized adult patients usually are given 100mg a day in divided doses, gradually increasing to 200mg daily if required. Adult outpatients are usually given 50-75mg a day in divided doses, increased to 150-300mg daily. Doses lower than 150mg may be given as a single dose at bedtime. Adolescents and elderly patients may be prescribed 10-30mg one to three times a day. In these cases, it is not usually necessary to exceed 100mg daily. Maintenance doses are normally from 75 to 150mg a day.

imipramine pamoate—Hospitalized patients may be started on 100-150mg a day and may be increased to 300mg daily. Dosages higher than 150mg a day may also be administered on a once-a-day basis after optimum dosage and tolerance has been determined. Adult outpatients may be started at 75mg daily and increased to 150mg a day. Maintenance dose for this drug in adults is usually 75-150mg a day. Elderly and adolescent patients should be given imipramine pamoate only when the daily dosage is established at 75mg or higher. For lower doses, these patients should take imipramine hydrochloride.

nortriptyline—For adults, 10-25mg three to four times a day (elderly people and adolescents may start with 10mg). The dosage may be increased as required to a maximum of 150mg daily in divided doses. The usual maintenance dose is 25-75mg a day.

protriptyline hydrochloride—Adults start with 5-10mg three to four times a day, and if necessary, dosage can be gradually increased to 60mg a day. Adolescents and older people are given lower doses, usually 5mg three times a day and increased gradually if necessary. In older people, the cardiovascular system should be monitored if the daily dose exceeds 20mg. With all users, when satisfactory improvement has been made, the dosage is usually reduced to the smallest amount that relieves symptoms. The last daily dose is normally given no later than 4 p.m.

maprotiline hydrochloride—Adults generally start with 25-75mg daily in three divided doses or as a single dose at bedtime. After two weeks, this may be increased gradually in 25mg increments as tolerated and required to a maximum of 225mg a day. Elderly and adolescent patients generally start with 25-30mg in three divided doses or at bedtime in a single dose, which can also be increased at a gradual rate.

amoxapine—Initial adult dose of 50mg is taken three times a day and may be increased to 100mg three times daily by the end of the first week of treatment if necessary, but sedation may occur at this level. When the effective dosage level is established, it can be given once a day at bedtime. Elderly and adolescent patients normally start at 25mg three times a day, which can be increased to 50mg three times daily. Between 100mg and 150mg a day is usually adequate for the elderly, but up to 300mg a day may be needed. Again, once the correct dose is determined it can be given at bedtime.

trazodone hydrochloride—Adults take 150mg in divided doses after meals or as a single dose at bedtime. Increments of 50mg a day can be added every three to four days (not to exceed a maximum dosage level of 600-800mg a day) as necessary. Maintenance dose is gradually reduced to an average level of 200-300mg a day. The elderly may start with

50-100mg daily in divided doses after meals or as one dose at bedtime.

trimipramine maleate—Initially, adults take 50-75mg daily in divided doses or as one dose two hours before bedtime. This may be increased as needed to a maximum of 300mg a day. The usual maintenance dose is 75-150mg daily. Elderly and adolescent patients start with 10-25mg three times a day with gradual increments allowed up to 100mg daily.

The prescribing physician will find a dosage level which is effective and doesn't cause side effects, and this can vary greatly from patient to patient. A tolerance to side effects quickly develops in most cases; they are also less of a problem if the dosage is increased gradually. This is especially important in the elderly, who may develop low blood pressure leading to dizziness and even fainting.

CONTRAINDICATIONS

Not recommended for patients recovering from heart block (irregular contraction of the heart) or a heart attack, or patients with mania. Not to be taken along with MAOIs, or for 14 days after taking MAOIs. Certain people are sensitive to these drugs and will exhibit side effects almost immediately. These people should not use TCAs.

CAUTION

These drugs should be used with caution when treating epileptics, because they lower the convulsive threshold. The smallest effective doses of these drugs are used because overdose can be very dangerous (although this is less of a problem with newer drugs such as trazodone). Many of these drugs cause some degree of sedation, which can affect a person's ability to drive a car or operate machinery. Caution is used for patients with diabetes, heart disease (especially if there is an irregular heart beat), liver disease, thyroid disease, psychotic conditions, closed-angle glaucoma, or difficulties with urination. Use of these drugs should not be discontinued abruptly. If a person has to be given general anesthesia, the chance of an irregular heart rate is increased. The safety of these drugs in pregnant women, nursing mothers, and very young children has not been established.

SIDE EFFECTS

The anticholinergic (chemical action that blocks the effect of the neurotransmitter acetylcholine) effects seen with antipsychotics can occur also with the use of these drugs. These include: dry mouth, blurred vision, constipation, and sweating. Hypotension (low blood pressure) leading to dizziness or fainting may also occur (especially in the elderly). Less commonly seen is urinary retention. Mania, schizophrenic excitement, and exacerbation of latent psychosis has been seen in susceptible people. The sedation these drugs can cause may be unpleasant. Cardiovascular effects normally occur only with overdose, but because many of these drugs can cause palpitations and affect the heart in other ways, a thorough cardiac history is usually taken before these drugs are prescribed. Agitation, fine tremors, hostility, skin rashes, itching, loss of appetite, diarrhea, nausea, confusion (particularly in the elderly), reduced sexual interest or impotence, edema (swelling) of the face and tongue, sensitivity to sunlight or bright light, insomnia, nightmares, headaches, ringing in the ears, and restlessness are also possible adverse side effects. Symptoms of overdose include drowsiness, stupor, coma, poor coordination, restlessness, agitation, muscle rigidity, and convulsions.

DRUG-DRUG INTERACTIONS

Because alcohol enhances the effects of these drugs, and vice versa, one should not drink while on these medications. Extreme sedation and even suicidal feelings could result. Antihypertensive drugs such as guanethidine monosulfate (Esimil, Ismelin) and clonidine (Catapres) can become less effective. Oral contraceptives may increase the effectiveness of these drugs, while antipsychotics can increase the plasma levels and the side effects. Barbiturates can decrease the effectiveness of these drugs. These drugs can increase the effects of vasoconstrictors such as epinephrine and norepinephrine (thereby raising blood pressure). It is potentially dangerous to combine TCAs with MAOIs.

DRUG-NUTRIENT INTERACTIONS

These drugs slow down the rate at which the stomach empties its contents into the intestines, which can cause constipation, especially in the elderly. Adding bulk to the diet in the form of whole grains (oatmeal and other whole-grain cereals, brown rice, whole-wheat breads) should alleviate the problem. Exercise is also beneficial. In cases of persistent constipation, the amount of fluid consumed in a day should be doubled. Bran can be added to the diet gradually, and fluid intake should be increased by at least 3/4 cup per teaspoon of bran.

Dry mouth is one side effect of these drugs. Too little saliva is secreted, reducing a person's ability to digest carbohydrates (saliva contains an enzyme that breaks down starches in the mouth to aid in their digestion) and making swallowing more difficult. The fiber of whole-grain products stimulates the flow of saliva and so should become an integral part of the diet. A shortage of saliva can also increase the risk of tooth decay and gum disease, so teeth should be brushed and flossed often, preferably after every meal.

These drugs may increase appetite and lead to weight gain.

THERAPEUTIC STIMULANTS

Many years ago, some people believed that stimulants could relieve depression. Unfortunately, these drugs had so many adverse side effects (insomnia, anxiety, anorexia) and had such high potential for tolerance and addiction, they caused more troubles in many cases than they cured (see Chapter Sixteen).

Today, the only types of problems treated with stimulants are attention-deficit disorders with hyperactivity, mainly in children. These drugs should be prescribed and monitored by a physician well-versed in the field.

GENERIC AND BRAND NAMES

methylphenidate hydrochloride *(Ritalin)*
pemoline *(Cylert)*

USES
methylphenidate hydrochloride—Attention-deficit disorders such as hyperactivity in children; also used to treat depression in the elderly and mild depression in adults, but its use in the latter two cases is now controversial.

pemoline—Attention-deficit disorders such as hyperactivity in children.

ACTION
Stimulates the central nervous system, but specifically how or at what site is unknown.

DOSAGE
methylphenidate hydrochloride—Adults usually take 20-30mg daily in divided doses 30-45 minutes before meals. Children over the age of six take 5mg two times a day (before breakfast and lunch) with gradual

increments of 5-10mg a week to a maximum of 60mg a day. The drug is usually discontinued for periods of time—often during school holidays—when learning is not as essential, in order to permit increased appetite and catch-up growth.

pemoline—One dose each morning, starting with 37.5mg a day, and gradually increasing by 18.75mg daily at one-week intervals until the effective dose is reached—usually 56.25-75mg. Maximum recommended dose is 112.5mg a day. Treatment for three to four weeks usually is necessary before significant benefits are seen.

CONTRAINDICATIONS

methylphenidate hydrochloride—Not recommended for children under the age of six, people with severe depression, and psychotic children (because it may exacerbate the symptoms).

pemoline—Not recommended for patients with liver disease.

CAUTION

methylphenidate hydrochloride—This drug can increase anxiety, tension and agitation, and may worsen glaucoma. It may also exacerbate tics in those already suffering from them or with a family history of Tourette's syndrome. Safety for use in pregnant women and nursing mothers has not been established. This drug can cause dependence in susceptible people, such as those with a history of alcoholism or drug dependency. This drug may induce seizures in patients who are prone to them, and also may increase blood pressure.

pemoline—Caution should be exercised in patients with impaired kidney function. Little information is available about safety during pregnancy, lactation, and for children under the age of six. This drug may exacerbate symptoms in psychotic children, and also may precipitate motor and phonic tics and Tourette's syndrome in susceptible patients when used over a long period of time. Emotionally unstable people may abuse this drug.

SIDE EFFECTS

methylphenidate hydrochloride—Insomnia is the most common side effect, but is usually controlled by reducing the dosage and omitting the afternoon dose. Other side effects include: nervousness, skin rashes, loss of appetite, nausea, dizziness, palpitations, headache, drowsiness, high blood pressure, changes in heart rate (up or down), stomachache, weight loss, anxiety, hallucinations, increase in pre-existing psychotic symptoms.

pemoline—Adverse reactions include depressed growth in children, weight loss, insomnia, impaired liver function, anorexia, nausea, stomachache, skin rash, and possible anemia. Central nervous system effects could include: Tourette's syndrome in susceptible people, hallucinations, abnormal movements of the tongue, lips, face, limbs, and eyes, mild depression, dizziness, headache, hyperexcitability, and worsening of glaucoma. This drug also lowers the threshold for seizures in patients who are prone to them.

DRUG-DRUG INTERACTIONS
methylphenidate hydrochloride—May decrease the effectiveness of the antihypertensive drug guanethidine monosulfate (Esimil, Ismelin). It may also increase the potency of common anticoagulants, anticonvulsants, the anti-inflammatory drug phenylbutazone (Butazolidin) and tricyclic antidepressants.

pemoline—Should not be taken within two weeks of using an MAOI as this can cause a hypertensive crisis.

DRUG-NUTRIENT INTERACTIONS
Therapeutic stimulants may reduce appetite and lead to weight loss and subsequent broad nutrient deficiencies. Pemoline should be taken after meals.

CHAPTER TWELVE
Antianxiety Agents

Antianxiety medications are probably the most widely known group of psychoactive drugs. Diazepam, more commonly known by the brand name Valium, was once the most-prescribed drug in this country. However, it began to receive some bad press (for the most part unjustified) and lost some of its popularity. This was largely due to the fact that people were abusing it and/or taking too much. Still, diazepam and the group of benzodiazepine antianxiety agents it belongs to—developed in the 1950s—are in common and constant use for the treatment of anxiety, panic and phobic attacks, seizures, insomnia, and withdrawal from the abuse of substances such as alcohol. These drugs may also be used pre-operatively to make the patient feel more at ease.

These medications produce calmness and relaxation, but of a different quality than the antipsychotics. They tend to be less sedating than the latter, but rather bring an anxious person back to a normal state of excitement. Again, it should be noted that these drugs do not cure—they simply alleviate symptoms. They do not usually help patients with severe personality disorders, affective disorders, schizophrenia or other symptoms of psychoses.

All have depressant effects on the central nervous system. They can be very sedating and even dangerous when combined with other CNS depressants such as alcohol. It is vital to stress that these drugs can be dangerous if abused in certain ways. It is hard to take enough of an antianxiety agent alone to cause death from overdose (with the exception of meprobamate), but in combination with alcohol or barbiturates, the results can easily be fatal. Many accidental deaths in this country have been caused by carelessly combining these minor tranquilizers with drink or other drugs. Antianxiety drugs can also cause dependence, and their prolonged use is not recommended. They should also not be stopped abruptly, since there can be some withdrawal symptoms. But all in all, when prescribed and monitored by a physician, they are relatively safe, and side effects are not that common. Many also have muscle relaxant and anticonvulsive properties, and can be used for epileptic seizures; clonazepam (Klonopin) is the drug of choice here. Chronic pain, especially where muscular tension is involved, is also relieved by the use of some antianxiety drugs. Lorazepam (Ativan) and oxazepam (Serax) are sometimes prescribed to treat akathisia, a motor disturbance causing extreme restlessness, which is a side effect from the use of antipsychotic drugs (see Chapter Thirteen).

Some drugs are long-acting and some are short-acting, which describes their period of effectiveness and how long they stay in the body.

Besides benzodiazepines, certain antihistamines are also used to treat anxiety, even though most of us think of them as a medication for allergies, rashes, itching, etc.

In cases where depression exists along with extreme anxiety, an antidepressant and an antianxiety agent may be simultaneously prescribed for a period of time, but again, this must be constantly supervised by a physician well-versed in the use of psychoactive drugs.

Although they have drawbacks, these drugs are far better than the sedative-hypnotics (barbiturates) that were previously used. These are extremely dangerous when combined with alcohol, cause heavier sedation, and are easily addictive. A tolerance to barbiturates quickly develops, and a patient is apt to start taking higher and higher doses— sometimes overdoses. Today, the main use of sedative-hypnotics is for the short-term treatment of acute insomnia.

Insomnia is often a symptom of severe anxiety. When it is the main one, the drugs of choice are flurazepam, triazolam or temazepam (benzodiazepines), chloral hydrate (a sedative-hypnotic), and diphenhydramine hydrochloride (an antihistamine). The latter two drugs are not listed in this section since they are used for insomnia, rather than full anxiety disorders.

A new drug being used experimentally, called buspirone (Buspar), is proving to be an effective antianxiety agent, with fewer side effects than many benzodiazepines. Future clinical use will provide more information concerning this drug.

The reasons why one might take an antianxiety agent differ widely. Sometimes people are given small, short-term doses of antianxiety agents for perfectly understandable reasons. A woman who finds her husband dead, a person whose house has just burned down, a father/mother of three who has just lost a job and has no savings, a person involved in a minor traffic accident, or someone going into major or minor surgery could all benefit from the calming effects of these drugs. On the other hand, more serious anxiety disorders may also be relieved in this way.

BENZODIAZEPINES

GENERIC AND BRAND NAMES

alprazolam *(Xanax)*
clorazepate dipotassium *(Tranxene)*
chlordiazepoxide *(Librium, Libritabs)*
diazepam *(Valium, Valrelease)*
*flurazepam *(Dalmane)*
halazepam *(Paxipam)*
lorazepam *(Ativan)*
oxazepam *(Serax)*
prazepam *(Centrax)*
*temazepam *(Restoril)*
*triazolam *(Halcion)*

*Manufactured as hypnotic agents;
usually not recommended for children

USES

These drugs are used to treat anxiety-related problems, panic and phobic symptoms, and insomnia. They are sometimes employed as an adjunct in alcohol withdrawal, and can also be used as anticonvulsants, muscle relaxants, and anesthetics.

ACTION

These drugs appear to reduce the activity of those areas of the brain responsible for emotion, and to increase the action of gamma-aminobutyric acid (GABA), the main inhibitory brain neurotransmitter. In the case of meprobamate, it has the same apparent action as other benzodiazepines, although its effects are more similar to barbiturates (though less potent).

USUAL DOSAGE

alprazolam—Initial dose is 0.25-0.5mg three times a day, which can be increased according to need, usually not to exceed a total daily dose of 4mg in divided doses. The elderly and debilitated are normally started on 0.125mg two to three times a day.

clorazepate dipotassium—7.5-60mg daily at bedtime or in two to three divided doses. The elderly and debilitated are normally given no more than 3.75mg initially.

chlordiazepoxide—For mild to moderate anxiety and tension, 5-10mg three to four times a day. For severe anxiety and tension, 20-25mg three or four times a day. Elderly and debilitated patients usually take as low a dose as possible to prevent over-sedation (5mg two to four times daily) and children may take 5-20mg daily in divided doses. The effectiveness of this drug for periods longer than four months has not been established.

diazepam—For anxiety, 2mg three times daily increased in cases of severe symptoms to 15-40mg daily in divided doses. Elderly and debilitated patients are given half these amounts. For children, 1-5mg given daily in divided doses is normally prescribed. For insomnia, 5-30mg are given at bedtime.

flurazepam—For insomnia mainly, 15-30mg before bedtime. For elderly and debilitated patients, 15mg is the usual dose.

halazepam—20-40mg three to four times daily. For the elderly and debilitated, usual dose is 20mg one to two times daily.

lorazepam—For anxiety, 1-4mg daily in divided doses, which can be increased to 10mg daily for severe anxiety. The elderly and debilitated start with 1-2mg daily, with the dose adjusted as needed. For anxiety-induced insomnia, 1-4mg as a single dose at bedtime.

oxazepam—For anxiety, 15-30mg three to four times a day, with dosage increased as needed to a maximum of 60mg twice daily in cases of extreme anxiety. The elderly and debilitated take 10-20mg three to four times daily.

prazepam—30mg (15mg for the elderly and debilitated) in divided doses. Usual dose range is 10-60mg daily. May also be given as a single dose at bedtime in 20mg amounts (less for the elderly and debilitated).

temazepam—Usual adult dose is 15mg a day, 30-60 minutes before bedtime. Elderly and debilitated patients start with 15mg and the dose is gradually increased until the individual effective level is determined.

triazolam—0.25-0.50mg is given 15 to 30 minutes before bedtime. 0.125-0.25mg is given in the same manner to elderly and debilitated patients.

CONTRAINDICATIONS

Some people are sensitive or allergic to these drugs and should not take them. If you have experienced a special sensitivity to alcohol or barbiturates, you may also have this problem with benzodiazepines. On the whole, pregnant women, nursing mothers, patients with severe respiratory problems, and those with a history of drug abuse should avoid taking these drugs unless a physician decides otherwise. These drugs are not normally used for patients with severe depression or psychotic disorders.

Additional information (where appropriate):

alprazolam—Safety not established for children under the age of 18.

clorazepate dipotassium—Not for children under the age of 9.

chlordiazepoxide—Not for children under the age of 6.

diazepam—Not for children under the age of six months.

flurazepam—Not for children under the age of 15.

halazepam—Not for children under the age of 18.

lorazepam—Not for children under the age of 12.

oxazepam—Not for children under the age of 6.

prazepam—Not for children under the age of 18.

temazepam—Not for children under the age of 18.

triazolam—Not for children under the age of 18.

CAUTION

Caution should be used in people with kidney and liver ailments, and in the elderly and debilitated. It is best not to take these drugs for a long period of time and never in quantities over the amount prescribed. Benzodiazepines, if abused, can cause physical and psychological dependence. However, they should not be stopped abruptly, since symptoms of withdrawal (which may occur from three to 10 days after cessation of use) can include nervousness, anxiety, agitation, insomnia, irritability, diarrhea, muscle aches, convulsions, and loss of memory. Benzodiazepine withdrawal is done by gradually reducing the dosage over a period of several days or weeks. Phenobarbital (a barbiturate) may be substituted, and then its dosage gradually reduced. Occasionally, these drugs produce "paradoxical reactions" in a small number of people susceptible to them. These patients become extremely agitated, hostile, anxious, or experience hallucinations. This is not common, however, since the majority of people are calmed down by these drugs.

Mental and physical abilities may be impaired while using these drugs, making driving a car or operating machinery hazardous.

SIDE EFFECTS

Possible adverse side effects include: drowsiness, confusion, dizziness, dry mouth, gastrointestinal disturbances, headache, unsteadiness, nausea, edema (swelling), nightmares, rashes, low blood pressure, difficulty in coordinating movements, and breathing problems. Less commonly seen are increased salivation, fatigue, depression, hypersensitivity reactions (like allergies), lethargy, apathy, light-headedness, body and joint pains, sweating, problems with vision, and irregular heart rate.

DRUG-DRUG INTERACTIONS

These drugs exacerbate the effects of alcohol and other CNS depressants. Overdose, serious illness, or death can result from these combinations. Anyone suspected of suffering from an overdose should be brought to a hospital emergency room—make sure to bring the bottle so the physician knows which drug was taken. Mild overdoses can cause drowsiness, mental confusion, and lethargy, while more serious cases result in poor muscle coordination, low blood pressure, deep sleep, and coma.

DRUG-NUTRIENT INTERACTIONS

Appetite may be increased, leading to weight gain, and if this happens the patient is placed on a balanced weight-loss diet. Since gastrointestinal disturbances—diarrhea, nausea, vomiting, and stomachache—may accompany the use of many of these drugs, it is best to take them with meals, especially for patients who suffer from these effects.

ANTIHISTAMINES

GENERIC AND BRAND NAMES

hydroxyzine hydrochloride *(Atarax, Durrax, Marax, Neucalm)*
hydroxyzine pamoate *(Vistaril, Hy-Pam, Vamate)*
diphenhydramine *(Benadryl)*

USES

Although the main use of antihistamine drugs is in the treatment of allergies, nausea, motion sickness, cough, itching, to relieve congestion, and as a local anesthetic, certain specific ones are beneficial in the treatment of anxiety.

hydroxyzine hydrochloride—Treatment of anxiety and tension associated with neurotic disorders. Effectiveness for periods of over four months has not been established.

hydroxyzine pamoate—Treatment of neuroses and emotional disturbances marked by anxiety, tension, agitation, apprehension, and confusion. It induces a calming effect in anxious, tense adults and also in anxious, hyperkinetic (overactive) children without impairing mental alertness. It is also used as an adjunctive therapy in alcoholics to ease anxiety and withdrawal symptoms. Effectiveness for periods of over four months of use has not been established.

diphenhydramine—Used as a mild antianxiety agent and sedative.

ACTION
Unknown at this time.

USUAL DOSAGE
hydroxyzine hydrochloride—25mg three to four times a day. Children up to six years of age, 30-50mg; children over the age of six, 50-100mg—all given daily in divided doses.

hydroxyzine pamoate—50-100mg four times daily; children over the age of six, 50-100mg daily in divided doses; children under the age of six, 50mg daily in divided doses.

diphenhydramine—25-100mg daily.

CONTRAINDICATIONS
Should not be used in the first trimester of pregnancy, by nursing mothers because its safety has not been established, or by people who are sensitive to these drugs.

CAUTION
Pregnant women are not advised to take these drugs, and they should be used with caution in patients with epilepsy, enlarged prostates, glaucoma, and liver disease. The ability to drive a car or operate machinery may be impaired.

SIDE EFFECTS
Possible adverse side effects include: impairment of mental and physical

abilities due to mild drowsiness, difficulty in urinating, dry mouth, blurred vision, headache, tremor, and gastrointestinal disturbances.

DRUG-DRUG INTERACTIONS

These drugs may increase the potency of meperidine (Demerol) and barbiturates, as well as alcohol.

DRUG-NUTRIENT INTERACTIONS

These drugs may be taken with a non-alcoholic beverage, but if gastrointestinal problems should occur, they may be taken with meals.

CHAPTER THIRTEEN

Antipsychotics

This group of drugs is among the most widely used in psychiatric practice, and contains a variety of generic choices. Although there can be many unpleasant side effects that accompany the use of these powerful medications, patients whose dosage level and length of treatment are carefully watched do not often encounter much trouble. In fact, the choice of drug to be prescribed often rests upon which one has the fewest side effects while at the same time providing the most benefits, which vary from person to person.

Chlorpromazine was the first modern antipsychotic agent to be discovered and used in the treatment of serious mental illnesses. Now other drugs in its chemical category—the phenothiazines—are also used, as well as the other classes of antipsychotics (which all resemble phenothiazines): butyrophenones, thioxanthenes, and dibenzoxazepines.

Since the 1950s these drugs have been used with great success to control the symptoms of schizophrenia and treat it and related psychoses, acute manic attacks, agitated depression (when used in conjunction with antidepressants), and organic brain diseases. They are also used for psychosis resulting from the abuse of certain drugs such as amphetamines. Many people with serious disorders are now able to lead more normal lives because of antipsychotic medications.

However, these medications have a down side that should be mentioned. If not prescribed and/or taken correctly, they can cause severe and sometimes long-lasting side effects. Also, the degree of sedation these drugs sometimes produce can be disturbing to both the patient and his or her family. For this reason, many physicians only use stronger drugs when absolutely necessary.

People taking antipsychotics should be aware of their side effects and take them only under the supervision of a qualified doctor.

GENERIC AND BRAND NAMES

Phenothiazines
chlorpromazine *(Thorazine)*
chlorpromazine hydrochloride (available under generic name)
fluphenazine hydrochloride *(Prolixin, Permitil)*
fluphenazine decanoate *(Prolixin Decanoate)*
mesoridazine *(Serentil)*
perphenazine *(Trilafon)*
thioridazine *(Mellaril, Mellaril-S)*
thioridazine hydrochloride (available under generic name)
trifluoperazine *(Stelazine)*

Dibenzoxazepines
loxapine succinate and loxapine hydrochloride *(Loxitane)*

Dihydroindolone
molindone hydrochloride *(Moban)*

Butyrophenones
haloperidol *(Haldol)*
haloperidol decanoate *(Haldol Decanoate)*

Thioxanthenes
chlorprothixene *(Taractan)*
thiothixene *(Navane)*

USES

This widely prescribed group of drugs is often called the *neuroleptics—*
which refers to any psychoactive drug that affects movement and
posture—to distinguish from other CNS depressants such as sedatives,
hypnotics, and opioids. Many neuroleptics are now used to treat chronic
or acute attacks of psychiatric illness.

Antipsychotic drugs are used to treat schizophrenia, paranoid disorders, acute attacks of mania, behavioral disturbances, psychosis associated with alcoholism, and organic brain disorders. They may be prescribed for anxiety if there is extreme agitation, and for various other
serious psychiatric problems. In cases of simple anxiety, they are not
commonly used because of their more pronounced side effects.

These medications control the symptoms of disturbed psychotic
patients. They can make schizophrenics more communicative and return them to a state of normalcy. The symptoms that respond best
include tension, hyperactivity, hostility, combativeness, delusions, hallucinations, anorexia and sleep disturbances.

Additional Information (where appropriate):
chlorpromazine and chlorpromazine hydrochloride—These are also useful in treating violent patients and extremely agitated elderly patients.

thioridazine and thioridazine hydrochloride—Prescribed for moderate to marked depression with anxiety, agitation in elderly patients, anxiety, depressed mood, and hyperactivity in children with behavioral problems such as impulsive actions, poor attention span, and extreme moodiness.

haloperidol—Can be used for the control of tics and vocalizations in both children and adults suffering from Tourette's syndrome.

ACTION
The precise mechanisms producing the therapeutic effects of these drugs is not known, but they affect all levels of the central nervous system, probably partly by inhibiting the actions of certain neurotransmitters.

USUAL DOSAGE
chlorpromazine and chlorpromazine hydrochloride—Oral doses of 10-25mg are given three times a day or in a single dose at bedtime. This may be raised if necessary after two or three days to 25-50mg three times daily, up to 800mg in psychotic situations until symptoms are controlled. In the elderly, a lower dosage is used and increments are gradual. For very agitated states in older people, no more than 25mg three times a day is normally used. In children up to five years of age, 5-10mg up to three times daily are given; in children 6-12 years, 1/3 to 1/2 the adult dose may be used.

Intramuscular injections are sometimes prescribed for acute psychoses in a hospitalized patient. 25mg may be given in a single dose and repeated in one hour if necessary. Oral doses (25-50mg three times a day) are then used once the patient calms down. Patients should lie down for 30 minutes after the injection, as it can be painful and may cause a rapid heart rate and drop in blood pressure.

Rectal suppositories of 100mg can be used every six to eight hours. 100mg of this drug given rectally are equivalent to 20-25mg injected, and 40-50mg in tablet form.

fluphenazine hydrochloride—For psychosis, 0.5mg-10mg are given in divided doses every six to eight hours. After maximum effect is achieved, the dose is gradually reduced. Older people are given reduced doses. For agitation, initially 1-2mg are given in the morning, increased as necessary to 4mg.

fluphenazine decanoate—12.5mg are given initially by intramuscular injection; after four to seven days, 12.5mg or more are given at intervals of 14-40 days, adjusted according to response. Gradual increases of 12.5mg are normally used, up to a maximum of 100mg.

mesoridazine—For schizophrenia, the initial dose is 50mg per day, adjusted accordingly. Optimum dose range is 100-400mg a day.

perphenazine—For moderately disturbed non-hospitalized patients, 4-8mg are given per day, reduced as soon as possible to the lowest effective dose, taken in divided doses. Hospitalized patients are given 8-64mg a day in divided doses. Intramuscular injections of 5-10mg are used for acute symptoms, followed if necessary by 5mg every six hours. Children receive the lowest adult dose.

thioridazine and thioridazine hydrochloride—For psychotic symptoms, 50-100mg are given three times daily with gradual increments if needed to a maximum of 800mg daily for up to four weeks. After symptoms are controlled, 100-200mg are given daily. No more than 300mg are given except for severe psychiatric conditions. For short-term treatment of moderate to marked depression with agitation, and for agitated, anxious and depressed symptoms in the elderly, 25mg are given three times a day. This can be increased to a maximum of 200mg daily for acutely disturbed patients.

For children (2-12 years), 0.5-3mg are given per kg of body weight per day. Children with moderately severe symptoms may take 10mg two to three times a day as a starting dose. Children hospitalized for a psychiatric condition may take 25mg two to three times a day as a starting dose. Dosage can be increased gradually until symptoms are controlled.

trifluoperazine—For psychoses, initially 2-5mg are given orally twice daily or 10mg daily in slow release form, adjusted upward after one week at three-day intervals to a maximum of 60mg, according to the response. For children (aged 6-12), initially 1-2mg are given once or twice a day, adjusted according to response, age, and body weight. Elderly patients with psychoses take doses in the lower range.

For acute symptoms, 1-2mg is administered initially by intramuscular injection followed by 1-2mg every four to six hours (rarely to exceed 10mg daily). For children, 1mg is administered once or twice a day. Once symptoms are controlled, the patient is returned to oral medication.

loxapine succinate and loxapine hydrochloride—Initial dose is 10mg two times a day (severely disturbed patients may need up to 50mg daily as an initial dose). Dosage may be increased over the first seven to 10 days until psychotic symptoms are under control. Usual maintenance level is 60-100mg a day.

molindone hydrochloride—Initially, 50-75mg a day are given, increased to 100mg daily after three or four days. This may need to be increased to 200mg daily in severe cases. Maintenance dose is 5-15mg, three or four times daily (for mild cases); 10-25mg three or four times daily (for moderate cases); and up to 200mg daily (for severe cases).

haloperidol—For moderate symptoms, 0.5-2.0mg are given orally two or three times a day. For severe symptoms, 3-5mg are given two or three times a day, up to 100mg for very severe cases. Once symptoms have been controlled, dose is reduced to lowest amount needed to be effective. For very agitated patients with severe symptoms, 2.5mg are administered by intramuscular injection, repeated as necessary. Children (aged 3-12) take lowest starting dose possible (0.5mg daily).

haloperidol decanoate—Dosage depends on previous oral dosage and physician's judgment.

chlorprothixene—For psychoses, 25-50mg are given three or four times a day, to be increased as needed. Very agitated patients can be given up to 600mg a day. Children (over six years) and the elderly with psychoses are given 10-25mg three or four times a day. For anxiety in adults, 30-45mg are given daily in divided doses.

thiothixene—For milder conditions, the starting oral dose is 2mg three times a day, increased to 5mg three times a day if necessary. For more severe conditions, the starting dose is 5mg two times a day. Usual optimal dose is 20-30mg daily. Increases up to a total of 120mg a day may be necessary in severe cases.

For rapid treatment of acute conditions, intramuscular injections of 4mg two to four times a day may be used. Dosage may be increased or decreased depending on response. An oral form replaces the injections as soon as possible.

CONTRAINDICATIONS

These drugs are not advised for people who are sensitive or allergic to them; who have blood, liver, kidney, or heart diseases; or who have severe depression. Safety for pregnant women and nursing mothers has not been established, so these drugs are rarely advised in such cases.

Additional Information (where appropriate):
fluphenazine hydrochloride—Not recommended for children.

fluphenazine decanoate—Not for children under 12, confused states, parkinsonism.

mesoridazine—Not for children under 12.

perphenazine—Not for children under 12.

thioridazine and thioridazine hydrochloride—Not for children under 2.

loxapine succinate and loxapine hydrochloride—Not for children under 16.

molindone hydrochloride—Not for children under 12.

chlorprothixene—Not for children under 6.

thiothixene—Not for children under 12.

CAUTION
These drugs can cause extreme sedation or drowsiness, especially in the beginning of their use, so driving a car or operating machinery can be dangerous. Older people may show more side effects and should take lower doses. Extreme caution should be taken in patients with glaucoma, epilepsy (can cause seizures), ulcers, or who have difficulty urinating. Withdrawal of the drug should be gradual and should also be watched, because a relapse of symptoms can occur as many as several weeks after stopping treatment. Other caution situations include: patients with Reyes' syndrome, cardiovascular disease, respiratory disease, parkinsonism, severe infections, kidney or liver disease, jaundice, and abnormally low-white-blood cell levels.

SIDE EFFECTS
These are the annoying aspects to these drugs—in fact, patients are often prescribed a particular type of antipsychotic drug because it is the one that does the job with the fewest or no side effects. Sedation and dizziness upon standing are common, but usually go away after prolonged treatment, as does an initial slowness in movement and reaction. Less common but more serious side effects include: jaundice (drug must be discontinued), breast enlargement, changes in blood pressure and hormone levels, and abnormal heart action.

Some of the most annoying side effects are the anticholinergic effects (which block the action of the neurotransmitter acetylcholine) such as dry mouth, blurred vision, and constipation, and the extrapyramidal effects, such as spasms of the neck muscles, rolling back of the eyes, restlessness, difficulty in swallowing, and other symptoms associated with Parkinson's disease. These can be treated with antiparkinsonism drugs such as benztropine mesylate (Cogentin). A late-appearing extrapyramidal effect called *tardive dyskinesia* can occur, causing tic-like, involuntary or semi-voluntary muscle movements, usually involving the tongue, face, and mouth muscles. It is more commonly seen in the elderly and with prolonged use.

Antipsychotic drugs can also cause faintness, palpitations, nasal stuffiness, and urinary retention. Body temperature may be poorly regulated, causing heat stroke upon exposure to high temperatures and hypothermia upon exposure to freezing weather (this is especially a danger in people over the age of 70). Fever, sexual dysfunction, an inability to sit still, skin rashes and sensitivity (making a person more prone to sunburn), gray-blue pigmentation of the skin, and in rare cases, cloudiness of the eye cornea causing vision problems have all been known to occur.

It seems strange to say that in spite of all these possible side effects, antipsychotic drugs are relatively safe, but they are. If the correct dosage is taken and medical supervision maintained, most patients have little trouble with these drugs, especially in cases of short-term use.

Differences between the antipsychotic drugs are less important than the patient's response and tolerance to the side effects. Selection of a drug is influenced by the amount of sedation required and the patient's susceptibility to extrapyramidal effects. However, specific drugs do have predominant characteristics and side effects, though again, this may not hold true for every patient.

The phenothiazine derivative drugs can be divided into three main groups (drugs of other chemical groups in the antipsychotic category tend to resemble the phenothiazines in Group III), although mesoridazine has a low incidence of side effects as compared to the other phenothiazines.

GROUP I:
chlorpromazine, chlorpromazine hydrochloride—Pronounced sedative effects, moderate anticholinergic and extrapyramidal effects.

GROUP II:
thioridazine, thioridazine hydrochloride—Marked anticholinergic effects, moderate sedative effects, fewer extrapyramidal effects than Group I.

GROUP III:
fluphenazine hydrochloride, perphenazine, trifluoperazine—Fewer sedative and anticholinergic effects than Groups I and II; more pronounced extrapyramidal effects than Groups I and II.

Additional Information (where appropriate):
chlorpromazine, fluphenazine hydrochloride, fluphenazine de-

canoate, perphenazine, thioridazine, thioridazine hydrochloride, trifluoperazine, haloperidol, chlorprothixene, and thiothixene—Apathy, paleness, nightmares, insomnia, depression, occasionally agitation, menstrual irregularities, weight gain. Rarely seen are impaired immunity and anemia.

fluphenazine hydrochloride—Fewer blood-pressure lowering effects.

fluphenazine decanoate—Extrapyramidal symptoms may appear a few hours after the dose has been given and continue for about two days but may be delayed. Pain, and occasionally redness, swelling, and nodules, can occur at the site of injection.

thioridazine and thioridazine hydrochloride—Vision problems may be seen rarely with higher doses, as can sexual dysfunction.

haloperidol—In rare cases, this drug interferes with liver function and causes an upset gastrointestinal tract.

chlorprothixene—Extrapyramidal effects are less frequent, but anticholinergic effects are seen more frequently.

DRUG-DRUG INTERACTIONS

In general, these drugs can: block the blood-pressure-lowering effects of guanethidine monosulfate (Esimil, Ismelin); show increased extrapyramidal effects if used with lithium, and metoclopramide hydrochloride (Ocatamide, Reglan) which is used to treat gastrointestinal disorders; become more potent if used with propranolol hydrochloride (Inderal, Inderide), an antihypertensive drug; increase the side effects seen with tricyclic antidepressants; make antiepileptic drugs such as phenytoin (Dilantin) less effective; increase the effects of anti-inflammatory drugs such as phenylbutazone (Butazolidin); and decrease potency of antiparkinsonism drugs such as levodopa (Larodopa, Sinemet). Antipsychotic drugs are not to be taken with alcohol or other CNS depressants; increased sedation and possible respiratory failure may result.

DRUG-NUTRIENT INTERACTIONS

These drugs should not be taken on an empty stomach as they can cause gastric distress. They may increase appetite and lead to weight gain.

When taken in high doses, some of these drugs may raise blood cholesterol levels, increasing the risk for heart disease. The diet can compensate for this effect to some extent. Limit cholesterol intake to 300mg a day, which means being careful about consuming foods such as red meat, eggs, and liver. The fat content of your diet should be reduced to 30 percent, consisting of equal parts of saturated fats (found in meat, fish and avocados), monounsaturated fats (found in fish and some vegetable oils such as olive oil), and polyunsaturated fats (found mainly in vegetables).

Chlorpromazine and related drugs may cause a riboflavin (vitamin B2) deficiency, resulting in dry skin around the nose and lips, cracks in the corner of the mouth, and a sore tongue. The eyes may burn and be more sensitive to light. Foods high in riboflavin, such as lean meats, dark green leafy vegetables, and enriched cereals and breads can be added to the diet, or a vitamin supplement can be taken daily.

If constipation is caused by using one of these drugs, it can be eased by increasing the bulk in the diet with larger servings of fiber-rich foods. Dry mouth and constipation can also be helped by doubling the amount of fluid taken in each day. If bran is used, it should be added to the diet gradually, and fluid increased by at least 3/4 cup per teaspoon of bran.

Additional Information (where appropriate):
loxapine succinate, loxapine hydrochloride, molindone hydrochloride, chlorprothixene, thiothixene—Drug-nutrient interactions not known at this time, but probably similar to the ones listed above for phenothiazines.

CHAPTER FOURTEEN

Lithium

Lithium is in a class by itself, and for many years its use was controversial. The reasons for its effectiveness are largely unknown, and its dosage must be carefully monitored. Despite this, it has saved the emotional lives of many people suffering from affective disorders—particularly bipolar illness (manic-depression) and acute mania.

Lithium is the lightest known metal, belonging to a group of alkali metals that includes sodium, potassium, rubidium, and cessium. Like these other metals, it does not occur as a free element, but as a salt. But just as sodium and potassium salts are usually referred to as sodium and potassium, lithium salts are called simply lithium. It is a trace element found in many chemical compounds, in naturally occurring minerals, in sea water, and in many sources of fresh water. In addition, small amounts of it have been discovered in certain plants and in animal tissues, although it is not known to play any physiological role in these organisms.

The use of lithium salts in the treatment of gout and urinary-tract stones can be traced back to the 1850s. In the early 20th century lithium bromide was used as a sedative and anticonvulsant, but eventually proved to be of no redeeming value. In the 1940s it was prescribed as a salt substitute for cardiac patients, but several deaths resulted and its administration was quickly stopped. However, in 1949, Dr. John F. Cade of Australia conducted a study concerning the effects of lithium in ten manic, six schizophrenic, and three chronically depressed patients. His results suggested that the substance had a specific antimanic effect.

Although to some degree the modern era of psychoactive drug treatment was initiated in 1949 with the discovery of the usefulness of lithium as a treatment for mania, it was rarely employed in clinical practice before 1970. Why? There are several theories to explain this unfortunate lag between discovery and application.

1. Its discovery in Australia had little impact on world psychiatry because the studies were reported only in local journals.
2. At the time, psychiatrists were not oriented toward the use of drugs to treat psychological problems.
3. Its toxic hazards discouraged its use.
4. Its benefits to a limited number of patients did not impress many psychiatrists.

GENERIC AND BRAND NAMES

lithium carbonate *(Eskalith, Eskalith CR, Lithane, Lithobid)*
lithium citrate *(Cibalith-S)*

USES

Lithium has been used increasingly over the past 15 years. Its main role is in the management of manic-depressive illness (see Chapter Seven). It has very little or no effect on people without psychiatric problems, and so is completely non-habit-forming. But for those with mood disturbances, it works in the following ways:

1. In cases of acute manic attacks, where the mania has reached psychotic proportions, lithium controls the problem in 70 percent of the patients treated. Because it may take several days to take effect, the person is also initially treated with antipsychotic drugs.
2. Lithium prevents or decreases the frequency and severity of manic and depressive episodes. However, it should be pointed out that since the drug removes the euphoric high of the manic stage, some patients dislike it because they feel the loss of those extreme "up" periods.
3. There is growing evidence that it can be helpful in the treatment of depression associated with bipolar illness. If this is firmly established, the implications will be far-reaching. Patients with bipolar disorder who are given TCAs for the depressive phase sometimes shift into a manic stage. If lithium is proved to be equal to the TCAs as an effective antidepressant, it will become the treatment of choice for depressed patients with bipolar disorder.
4. The drug has not yet been approved to treat unipolar depressive patients, although some evidence shows that it works as effectively as imipramine in preventing recurring episodes. Lithium does not appear to relieve acute depression.
5. Some people have reported that certain schizophrenics respond to lithium treatment. Why this should be so is not known, but there is

the chance that they are only reacting well to the drug because they have been misdiagnosed—they are really suffering from manic depression or an affective disorder with schizophrenic-like symptoms and not from schizophrenia.

It is important to remember that it is the manic stage of bipolar illness that responds best to lithium, and that it is not a cure for bipolar disorder. It simply prevents or limits future mood-swing episodes. The main limitation it has is the narrowness of the range between the correct, therapeutic dose and a toxic dose. This is why the level of lithium in the patient's blood must be constantly checked.

Although its use for children is very controversial, it is sometimes employed in the management of disorders marked by episodic changes in mood and behavior that resemble bipolar illness in adults. Mixed results have been reported when it is prescribed to treat premenstrual syndrome (PMS), drug and alcohol abuse syndromes, episodic aggression or anger, and anorexia nervosa. All in all, its main benefit is seen in the treatment of mania and the control of bipolar illness, to prevent recurrent attacks.

Manic-depression can disrupt a person's entire life. At this point, there is no other treatment that is as effective as lithium in dealing with bipolar disorders. Some reports cite a 70 percent improvement rate, which is significant by any standards.

ACTION

Lithium appears to cause the brain to use the catecholamine neurotransmitters more efficiently. It has no discernible effects on illness-free people. It is not a sedative, depressant, or euphoriant. Its action as a mood stabilizer is not fully understood, although effects on the brain cell membranes are suspected. It inhibits the release of norepinephrine and dopamine by the nerve terminals, but not the release of serotonin. It affects the distribution of sodium, calcium, and magnesium within the brain, and alters the mind's use of glucose (its main energy source). It reduces the activity of certain nerve cells in the brain, which may contribute to the manic state.

USUAL DOSAGE

When lithium is administered, the intention is to produce a particular concentration in the blood. It is this concentration that is important, and not the amount of medication given daily. If the concentration in the blood is too low, there will be no beneficial effects; if it is too high, side effects can appear. To regulate the dose, the patient is started at a low level for a few days. A blood sample is then taken to determine the status, and the dose is increased as needed. This means initially the patient must have a blood test each time the dose is increased. As the patient's response to lithium becomes regulated and the blood level stabilizes, tests can be conducted at less frequent intervals.

Doses of 300-2400mg of lithium carbonate are given daily, adjusted to achieve a blood plasma concentration of 0.6 to 1.2 milli-equivalents of lithium ions per liter of blood in a sample taken twelve hours after the preceding dose on the fourth or seventh day of treatment; samples are taken weekly until the dosage has remained constant for four weeks, and then monthly thereafter. Daily doses are usually divided; sustained-release preparations (such as Lithobid) are normally given twice daily. In the case of lithium citrate, the same procedure is followed except that 600mg are given twice daily, adjusting the dose until a plasma concentration of 0.6 to 1.2 milli-equivalents per liter is achieved.

In the initial stages of treatment for acute mania, supplementary doses of antipsychotic agents are usually advised, since it takes a few days for the drug to exert its effects. But high doses of any psychoactive drug may be dangerous when combined with lithium.

Reduced doses of lithium will be required in the elderly to achieve the same plasma levels, and dosage adjustments may be needed if the patient does heavy physical work or excessive exercising, both of which cause significant sweating and increase plasma levels of the drug.

CONTRAINDICATIONS

Heart patients are not advised to take lithium salts, especially if they are on low sodium diets. Such a diet prevents the excretion of the drug by the kidneys and increases the amount retained in the body. Plasma levels in excess of 1.5 milli-equivalents of lithium per liter may be toxic. Toxic effects can include tremor, unsteadiness and difficulty in coordinating movements, difficulty in speaking, rapid eye movements, kidney failure and convulsions. Patients with poor kidney function should not take lithium for the same reason—the inability to excrete it. It should not be used by pregnant women, especially during the first three months when it may cause birth defects, by nursing mothers, or given to young children.

CAUTION

Thyroid function should be watched, as cases of hypothyroidism have occurred. Adequate sodium and fluid intakes should be maintained to prevent a harmful build-up of the drug. Patients taking diuretics causing the loss of either potassium or sodium should be carefully monitored.

Long-term or high-dose use of lithium can cause kidney damage; patients are kept on the lowest possible maintenance doses.

SIDE EFFECTS

Lithium therapy is associated with a short-term increase in the excretion of sodium, potassium, and water; this effect does not last beyond 24 hours. In the subsequent four to five days of lithium treatment, the excretion of potassium becomes normal, but sodium is retained and can lead to both edema (swelling) and weight gain. These latter effects usually disappear after a few days, but weight gain can continue. Intense thirst and very frequent urination are often seen, but usually only persist in the early stages of therapy. Other side effects include vomiting, diarrhea, and fine tremor.

An overdose or build-up of lithium causes blurred vision, increased gastrointestinal disturbances (vomiting, diarrhea, and anorexia), and increased CNS problems (mild drowsiness, sluggishness increasing to giddiness with poor coordination of movements, tremor, and difficulty in speaking).

DRUG-DRUG INTERACTIONS

Diuretics causing sodium depletion such as thiazides increase blood plasma levels of lithium, as do indomethacin (Indocin), phenylbutazone (Butazolidin), ibuprofen (Motrin), and piroxicam (Feldene). Aminophylline (Aminophyllin, Mudrane, Somophyllin), and sodium bicarbonate increase lithium secretion, so decreasing its effectiveness. Haloperidol (Haldol) and the phenothiazine group of antipsychotic drugs increase the risk of tremor and other CNS disturbances.

DRUG-NUTRIENT INTERACTIONS

Lithium can cause gastrointestinal distress and weight gain. Patients on the drug should not be on sodium-restricted diets, as low blood sodium levels can enhance lithium's action by decreasing its excretion, resulting in a toxic build-up of the drug. In many people, a toxic effect, generally mild, will occur two to four hours after taking the drug, when it reaches its maximum concentration in the bloodstream, but people on very restricted sodium diets may suffer from more severe toxic reactions at this time.

PART THREE

DRUGS THAT CAUSE ILLNESS

INTRODUCTION:
Abusing the Mind and Body with Drugs

Drugs—even therapeutic drugs—can harm body and mind as much as or more than they help if used incorrectly or deliberately misused. The therapeutic benefits of a medication for treating anxiety, such as diazepam (Valium), can be reversed if the person for whom the drug is prescribed takes too much too often. This can lead to chemical dependence and an uncomfortable period of withdrawal. Other psychoactive agents, such as phencyclidine (PCP), heroin, and cocaine, have virtually no therapeutic value and their abuse can poison the brain and body.

People who take any type of drug for "fun" and not because a doctor prescribes it, or who take too much of a prescribed drug, are seriously endangering their health. Drug abuse is not a minor problem in our society. The statistics are sobering:

- Over one-third of young adults in this country use illicit drugs of some type.
- 22 million Americans have tried cocaine and 5 million currently use it.
- Over 90 billion dollars a year change hands in drug trafficking and manufacture.
- Americans pay over 40 billion dollars a year for lost productivity, accidents, and treatment services related to drug abuse.
- 16 percent of drivers arrested for unsafe driving, if a recent California study is representative, are under the influence of marijuana.
- The U.S. Armed Forces publicly acknowledge that drugs have had a negative impact on our defense capabilities.

Why do people abuse drugs? First of all, they offer pleasurable sensations, enhance intimacy, loosen inhibitions, and dampen anxiety—at least in the early stages of use. Many drug users say they have gained psychological and spiritual insights while under the influence of drugs. Peace of mind can be temporarily achieved, and that aspect appeals to people suffering from chronic depression, or who are living in a depressing socioeconomic environment.

But drug abuse is poisoning, pure and simple. Almost any drug will produce toxic qualities if taken frequently and/or in high enough doses. There are miserable side effects. Even worse, there can be long-term damage. Even a partial account of long-term effects related to various drugs is chilling. Glue-sniffing, which can have devastating effects on the kidneys and cell membranes of the brain, has also been linked to several forms of leukemia. Cocaine can weaken the heart, and amphetamines may permanently damage the brain. Chronic use of cocaine, amphetamines or narcotics often leads to severe malnutrition, with resulting vulnerability to disease and infection. Marijuana can damage the lungs and respiratory system. Drugs that are injected carry the risk of hepatitis, endocarditis (inflammation of the heart's lining and valves), and the deadly disease AIDS. Cocaine, if sniffed ("snorted") frequently, can destroy nasal passages, and cocaine or crack smoking can cause serious respiratory ailments.

In many cases, previously existing psychological problems can be brought out or exacerbated by drug abuse—and sometimes the drugs *cause* mental imbalance. Marijuana smokers often experience panic attacks or spells of paranoia. Toxic psychosis, which resembles schizophrenia and can last for several weeks to months, is regularly seen in those who use cocaine and amphetamines heavily. More profound drug-induced psychosis can be caused by the use of hallucinogens such as LSD or PCP. LSD users are vulnerable to "flashbacks"—a repeat of psychedelic experiences up to a year or more after drug use has ceased.

Even short-term temporary effects of drug use can be disastrous. Drugs affect judgment and performance, short-term memory, coordination, motor skills and perception. When drug use is combined with occupational or recreational activity, it causes accidents—automobile accidents, industrial accidents, skiing accidents, boating accidents, swimming accidents, and on and on. Hallucinogenics cause perhaps the most bizarre accidents of all. Users of LSD or other hallucinogens have been known to try to stop moving cars with their bare hands or to jump out of windows thinking they could fly. And drugs which raise body temperature, such as PCP, have often inspired users to go for swims— with the result that almost half of all PCP deaths are from drowning.

Drug use can damage or disintegrate social and marital relationships, cause estrangement between parents and children, and take the place of normal social activities. Sex, which is sometimes initially improved by drug use, is eventually pushed out of the picture completely. Sexual feelings, which may be enhanced initially by drug use, eventually lose their importance to the drug user as his life revolves increasingly around his need for drugs. Some drugs actually diminish sexual desire, even initially. In fact, the need to buy and use drugs often takes the place of everything else. Chronic crack smokers may sit around all day in "crack houses," surrounded only by "drug buddies," never seeing the sunlight. Disheveled, sick, and malnourished, the chronic drug abuser is often a tragic and pitiful sight.

Pregnant women can damage not only their own bodies, but also the bodies of their children, through drug abuse. Some chemicals, which seem to have little or no negative effect on the mother, may be extremely dangerous for the developing infant. Low birth weight is one problem commonly seen among babies whose mothers have misused drugs during pregnancy. Low birth weight is a major cause of infant death, increases the risk of infant illness, and has been connected to mental and physical handicaps, learning disorders, and behavior problems.

Fetal damage is not limited to low birth weight. When used during pregnancy, many drugs can result in gross malformations of the child's brain and body. Studies on the effects of cocaine during pregnancy, for example, show that the drug can interfere with blood flow to the fetus' brain, causing strokes and other types of brain damage.

Fetal addiction is another complication. Hospital workers say there is nothing sadder than seeing a newborn infant "withdraw" from the drugs his or her mother has been taking.

Drugs may also be transmitted through the mother's breast milk to the child, causing additional damage to the developing infant of a nursing mother.

DRUGS OF ABUSE

The drugs that are most often abused fall into the following categories:
- *Opioids*—heroin, morphine, methadone, opium
- *Depressants*—barbiturates, barbiturate-like hypnotics, sedatives
- *Stimulants*—amphetamine, amphetamine-like substances, cocaine (freebase, crack and cocaine hydrochloride)
- *Hallucinogens*—LSD, mescaline, psilocybin, etc.
- *Phencyclidines*—PCP, ketamine, PCP analogs (drugs similar in structure)
- *Cannabinoids*—marijuana, hashish, hash oil
- *Inhalants and volatile substances*—acetone, benzene, ethyl acetate, nitrous oxide, butyl nitrate, etc.
- *Designer drugs*—analogs of hallucinogenic amphetamines (MDA, MDMA), hallucinogens (DMT), opiates (3-methyl fentanyl, MPPP), phencyclidine (PCE, PCC) and methaqualone (mecloqualone)

Opioids are also called narcotic analgesics and are used medically to relieve pain. This category includes morphine and other alkaloids of opium. Abusers take them for the drowsy, euphoric state they induce, giving a dream-like sense of well-being and relaxation. On the street they go by the names "horse," "dope," "junk," and "H."

Depressants are exactly what their name implies; they depress excitable tissues at all levels of the brain. They include central nervous system (CNS) depressants, such as antianxiety drugs and sleep aids, and are sometimes called "solid booze" because their effects (particularly the barbiturates) are similar to alcohol. The street names for barbiturates are "downers," "reds," "barbs," and "yellow jackets"; for methaqualone they are "ludes," "sopor," and "lemons."

Stimulants excite the CNS, and produce euphoria, hypersensitivity, insomnia, and appetite suppression. They relieve fatigue and induce feelings of power. The aftermath of their use is the "crash" caused by the exhaustion of the CNS—panic, paranoia, nervousness, and increased appetite. The higher the high, the lower the low, so users must take more of the drug to get "up" again. This group includes all amphetamine-like substances, and cocaine in its many forms. Street names for cocaine include "coke," "snow," "toot," "flake," and "lady"; for amphetamines they are "uppers," "speed," "bennies," "black beauties," "dex," "meth," and "crank."

Hallucinogens produce hallucinations of sight, sound, smell, touch, and taste. This group includes LSD, mescaline, and psilocybin. These are natural or synthetic agents that can produce great changes in the mind, causing abnormal thinking from the massive disruption of normal brain processes. Street names include "acid," "sunshine," "microdots," "blotter" (LSD), and "buttons" (psilocybin).

Phencyclidines, of which the major drug is PCP, are related pharmacologically to hallucinogens and have somewhat similar effects, although there are different symptoms of tolerance and withdrawal. These agents offer a floating feeling, and a sense of detachment from one's surroundings. Their use can lead to violence and psychosis. They are known on the street as "peace pills," "angel dust," and "killer weed."

Cannabinoids, such as marijuana, hashish, and hash oil, are derived from the cannabis sativa plant. Their active ingredient, delta-9 tetrahydrocannabinol (THC), produces an intoxicated state, with an altered sense of time and space, euphoria, and at high doses, some hallucinations. These drugs can also cause excitability, or sleep. The street names for such drugs are "grass," "weed," "reefer," "joints," "herb," "pot," and "hash."

Inhalants and volatile substances include solvents widely used in cleaning compounds, aerosol sprays, fuels, and glues, as well as inhalants such as nitrous oxide and butyl nitrate. They cause altered states of consciousness, lightheadedness, and confusion associated with the general depression of brain function. On the street, many are simply known as "glue." Nitrous oxide may go by the names "laughing gas" and "nitrous," and the nitrates are often called "poppers," "snappers," "rush," and "bolt."

Designer drugs are a new and often dangerous category of chemicals that have been "doctored" in underground laboratories in such a way that makes them legal or significantly more potent. By changing some small parts of a drug's chemical structure, a chemist can make a new drug with the same or stronger effects and action than the original compound. Many drugs have designer copies. The opiate substitutes such as "fixed" fentanyls and meperidines have resulted in death from overdose, or in the latter case, a permanent state of Parkinson's disease caused by toxic chemical by-products.

HISTORY AND CONTROLS

Drug use has a long and sometimes surprising past. Ritual opium use has been traced to Greece and Cyprus in 2000 B.C. The ancient Aztecs used the hallucinogens of ololiuqui (similar to LSD), peyote, and marijuana. The fortunes of early New World merchants were increased by trading opium. And after the Civil War, doctors began prescribing opium-based concoctions for everything from headaches to skin rashes. Heroin, a morphine derivative, was sold legally at the turn of the century in drugstores, mail-order catalogs, and by traveling salesmen. At that time, it was estimated that one in 400 Americans used opiates regularly. Cocaine first became popular around the same time, and one pharmaceutical firm sold at least 15 products—from cigarettes to skin salve to face powder—laced with the drug.

But in the early 1900s, the rise of drug addiction and violent crimes associated with drug abuse began to frighten the general public. The U.S. banned the import of opium in 1909. In 1914, the Harrison Act placed controls on the use and sale of potentially dangerous drugs.

Today, with a new generation of drug users and ever-increasing problems, all regulations concerning the use of drugs for illicit consumption are covered under the Comprehensive Drug Abuse Prevention and Control Act of 1970. Title II of this legislation is more familiarly known as the Controlled Substances Act. In it, drugs are categorized into Schedules I, II, III, IV, or V. Persons convicted for possession and trafficking in drugs listed under Schedules I and II (such as PCP, cocaine, and narcotics) receive the most severe legal penalties.

THE ROAD TO DEPENDENCY

Drug abuse is the compulsive use of a psychoactive substance to the point where it endangers mental and physical health. It is often an uncontrollable, irrational use that seizes the life of the user and controls his every move. Even people who can function normally while taking drugs have a problem—many of them would fall to pieces if the drugs were taken away.

Drugs affect the pleasure centers of the brain, and different drugs stimulate different centers, producing varying effects. Once in the bloodstream, drugs go almost everywhere in the body, but are effective only where they find receptors. In the central nervous system, most drugs head for the synapses (the junctions between cells in the neural pathways along which brain signals travel). Not all drugs can easily cross the blood brain barrier, which is made up of the lining of capillaries in the brain that supply the brain with blood (see Figure 3). Unfortunately, the system is far from perfect: penicillin has a hard time getting across, but heroin gets an easy ride.

FIGURE 3 The Blood-Brain Barrier

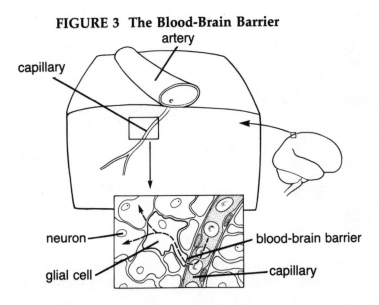

Brain signals, which are basically electrical impulses, often must wait to move until the chemical messengers called neurotransmitters stored at the synapses are released, flooding the gap, and allowing the signals to pass across. Drugs can stimulate or inhibit the release of neurotransmitters or keep them from being reabsorbed once they are used. Cocaine, for example, appears to stimulate the brain to release the neurotransmitters dopamine, serotonin, and norepinephrine, causing overstimulation and subsequent brain exhaustion. In addition, it blocks the return of neurotransmitters to the neurons for reuse. Figures 4 and 5 show how cocaine disturbs the flow and re-uptake of dopamine, nor-epinephrine, and serotonin. Eventually, the brain becomes depleted of these chemicals and needs cocaine for stimulation.

The abuse potential of any drug can be determined by pharmacological tests done on animals. Some drugs are more likely to lead to dependence than others. Psychological dependency is defined as a state where the user believes the drug is needed for maintaining his feelings of well-being or normalcy. Physical dependency occurs when the body's cells are so changed by constant exposure to the drug that they become incapable of functioning properly when deprived of it. Cocaine, once thought to cause only psychological dependency (which can be uncomfortable enough), may now be classed in both categories, because repeated use changes the nature of the brain cells so that they crave the drug.

FIGURE 4   **FIGURE 5**

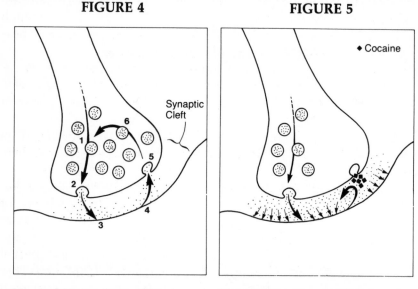

Normal Neurotransmitter   **Neurotransmitter Release and**
Release and Re-uptake   **Re-uptake Disturbed by Cocaine Use**

1. *Manufacture of neurotransmitter in the terminal button and movement toward the edge of the neuron;*
2. *Release of neurotransmitter into the synaptic cleft;*
3. *Neurotransmitter binding to receptor sites on the synaptic membrane of the next neuron in order to pass the message;*
4. *Release of neurotransmitter from receptor sites into the synaptic cleft after the message has been passed;*
5. *Re-uptake of neurotransmitter into the synaptic button;*
6. *Recycling of neurotransmitter for future use.*

Cocaine causes the increased release of neurotransmitter into the synaptic cleft, eventually draining the neuron of neurotransmitter. There is increased binding to receptor sites, and blocked re-uptake of neurotransmitter.

Tolerance, which develops rapidly with certain drugs such as barbiturates, means that more and more of the drug is craved or needed to produce the initial effect. In some cases, this leads to a dangerous situation, because a large amount of the drug is required by chronic users, while only a little more can cause overdose and possibly death.

Withdrawal from long-term drug abuse can be a painful and sometimes life-threatening process. In the case of barbiturates, the brain combats the drug's messages to "slow down" by causing the neurotransmitters to release a "stay alert" signal to the affected nerve tracts and brain nucleii. But when the drugs are suddenly stopped, the brain's "stay alert" messages continue to flow in abundance. This phenomenon is called rebound. The brain becomes hypersensitive, and with no external sedatives to stop this stimulation, the user goes through withdrawal, with symptoms ranging from discomfort and nervousness to extreme agitation and sometimes fatal convulsions.

The word "addiction" is rarely used anymore, and has been exchanged for the term "dependence." Both words refer to an extreme form of compulsive drug use, where the drug becomes the central part of life.

In addition to the adverse effects of drug abuse already mentioned, all drug abusers face special dangers which in many cases can cost them their lives.

Overdose can result not only when too much of one drug is used, but also when two similar drugs are taken together. This could be, for example, two depressants, or a depressant with alcohol, or a depressant with an opioid. Because the tolerance to many drugs increases rapidly, users may be tempted to take similar substances to enhance the effect of their drug of choice. Because drug abusers rarely pay attention to dose levels, the cumulative effects of all the drugs they take at one time can reach lethal levels. Overdose can also result when a person thinks he is taking one drug and it is really another, or when the drug strength has been artificially boosted (as in the case of the new "designer" opiates).

Illicit drugs can affect the potency of necessary prescription medications, rendering them in some cases much less effective. Barbiturates reduce the potency and duration of action of many medicines by speeding up metabolism in the liver. Antifungal agents, anticoagulants, some cortisone drugs, and digitalis are all affected by drugs of abuse.

Certain users are at special risk when they take illegal drugs. These people include:

• Heart patients, who are in danger from drugs that produce stress, such as hallucinogens or stimulants, and from drugs that cause stressful withdrawals. Smoking marijuana raises the heart rate and can precipitate angina pectoris.

• Pregnant women, who should stay away from all types of drugs, including alcohol. Miscarriage, premature births, fetal defects, and learning disabilities can be caused by drug abuse. Nursing mothers should remember that most chemicals pass into breast milk and can further damage the child's development.

• Epileptics, whose seizures can be caused or exacerbated through drug abuse. In addition, anticonvulsant drugs should not be taken with depressants. The effects of these medications are intensified, and seizures become likely during withdrawal.

• Adolescents, whose rapidly growing bodies are especially vulnerable to the toxic effects of chemicals. Drugs can cause disruptions in hormonal changes taking place at this time. Infantile self-involvement, poor learning habits, and delayed maturation are all possible adverse behavioral effects.

AIDS (Acquired Immune Deficiency Syndrome) is a new and vicious threat to intravenous-drug users, who are in one of the two highest risk categories for contracting the often fatal disease caused by the HIV virus. AIDS prevents the immune system from protecting the body against certain previously rare "opportunistic" tumors and infections, such as Kaposi's sarcoma (a type of cancer) and *Pneumocystis carinii pneumonia*. Symptoms of AIDS, which was at first thought to be restricted in this country to male homosexuals, include diarrhea, fever, weight loss, swollen glands, and severe fatigue. It is believed that at least 50 percent of those tested positive for the virus will die from it. The ailment is spread among IV-drug users by sharing needles.

In the following chapters, we will be looking at specific drugs of abuse in greater detail, describing their actions, adverse effects, and the ways in which abusers may be helped through treatment programs.

CHAPTER FIFTEEN

STIMULANTS:
Cocaine and Crack

Cocaine is taken into the body in three ways. Injection is rare, unless the drug is combined with an opioid such as heroin or meperidine—a process known as "speedballing." Many deaths, including that of comedian John Belushi, are linked to this method of abuse. But most users either "snort" the drug intranasally or smoke it as freebase, or as a new and highly addictive pre-prepared freebase product called "crack." The drug is much more addictive and harmful when it is smoked, because it reaches the brain in higher doses and in a matter of seconds, as opposed to several minutes when it is snorted. But no matter how it is taken, cocaine harms the mind and body.

Although Sigmund Freud described the horrors of cocaine-induced psychosis in 1884 (while he was using the drug), and for centuries certain South American Indian tribes have been chewing coca leaves to relieve fatigue and enhance ceremonial rites, cocaine abuse is the major drug problem of today. More than 22 million Americans have tried cocaine and five million currently use it. While opiate addiction and arrests have remained at a constant level for the past 15 years, and marijuana and amphetamine use has dropped, the use of and arrests for cocaine rise every month.

The cost to this country in terms of reduced work productivity, drug treatment, and cocaine-related crimes is staggering. Cocaine addicts come from all walks of life, but because of the drug's high cost ($100 or more for a gram), addicts are often economically prosperous people who hold positions of significant power and authority. Unfortunately, the drug has been associated with glamorous industries and lifestyles, such as show business, professional athletics, and Wall Street finance.

The tragic misconception that has accompanied the rise of cocaine abuse since the 1970s is that it does not lead to drug dependency or addiction. It was first believed that the addiction was psychological, in a mild sense—not physiological. We know now from increasingly frightening evidence that cocaine is one of the most addicting substances known to mankind. When laboratory animals are given unlimited access to cocaine, they prefer it to food, sex, and everything else, and they will use it until it kills them. They become obsessed with the drug and will press a bar hundreds of times to try and obtain another dose. Human beings seem to be no different. The addiction is both psychological and physical—cocaine appears to cause profound changes in the basic chemistry of the human brain.

Like most drugs, cocaine use was at first accepted by society. U.S. President Ulysses Grant used cocaine on the advice of his publisher, Samuel Clemens (better known as Mark Twain), in his last years while writing his memoirs. And Freud extensively chronicled the many "benefits" of cocaine use. Its use first became popular in the U.S. in the late 19th century. At that time, one pharmaceutical company sold at least 15 products laced with cocaine, including cigarettes, skin salve, and face powder. When Coca-Cola was first released, it contained small amounts of cocaine. (Today's Coca-Cola is still made in part from coca leaves, but the cocaine has been removed.)

By the 1920s, drug use and the violent crimes associated with it started to concern society. Cocaine abuse went underground, confined mainly to musicians and avant-garde actors and artists. But the mid-1970s marked its re-emergence, and its use has risen steadily since then. It has now become a problem for everyone in society—whether they use it, or suffer because of others who do.

Basically, cocaine is a stimulant. It is used to produce euphoria, feelings of power and intellect, increased energy, reduced fatigue, and appetite suppression. People initially feel they can work better and for longer hours while taking the drug. However, with chronic use the drug so disturbs thought processes and attention span that professional and social lives eventually suffer, even collapse. The high cost of this addiction can bankrupt even a wealthy man over a period of time.

Cocaine users build up a tolerance to the drug, necessitating larger and larger amounts to achieve the same "high" they had initially. They reach a point where they don't feel the euphoric state anymore, but rather need to use large quantities of the drug just to feel somewhat normal.

Cocaine hydrochloride is a white, crystalline powder (actually a salt) produced from cocaine base, a product of coca paste, which comes from the coca plant that grows abundantly in the eastern Andes mountains of South America. The major sources of cocaine are growers and distributors in the South American countries of Bolivia, Peru, and Colombia. The drug is available here at about 30-40 percent purity. In this form, cocaine is "cut" or watered down with sugars such as lactose or other amphetamine-like stimulants, and is sniffed through the nose.

Freebasing (the first term used to describe cocaine smoking) was introduced in the late 1970s. Freebase is formed by mixing cocaine hydrochloride with a strong alkali and ether, and then evaporating it and removing the hydrochloride. The conversion to freebase does two things: purifies the highly adulterated cocaine and converts it to a form that vaporizes more readily when smoked. Because this process involves the use of volatile chemicals such as ether, and elaborate paraphernalia such as acetylene or butane torches, it is dangerous and complicated. Explosions have resulted and users have been burned.

Unlike cocaine manufactured for smoking using the older freebasing method, crack—which first became popular in the early 1980s—is the "street" name given to freebase cocaine that has been processed differently. Ammonia or baking soda and water are added to cocaine hydrochloride and heated to remove the hydrochloride, as opposed to the more volatile method of processing that uses ether. The process used to convert cocaine hydrochloride to crack does not necessarily result in the elimination of all the hydrochloride, sodium bicarbonate and fillers and impurities in the cocaine. (The term "crack" probably refers to the cracking sound that is heard when the mixture is smoked, presumably due to the sodium bicarbonate.)

Crack is sold in small vials and is in the form of small, ready-to-smoke, creamy-colored chunks. It can be used in a special pipe or sprinkled over cigarettes containing tobacco or marijuana.

In 1986, a spokesperson for the National Cocaine Hotline estimated that one million Americans in 25 states around the country had tried crack. Most abusers at that point were males between the ages of 20 and 35. Because crack appears less expensive than cocaine hydrochloride (vials often sell for $10 to $20), it caught on quickly in inner-city areas among people in lower socioeconomic groups. The problem has now spread to all areas of the population. In reality, because of its highly addicting nature, crack is as expensive or more so than regular cocaine. A user must buy vial after vial to maintain his "high."

COCAINE HYDROCHLORIDE

METHOD OF ACTION

Cocaine can be absorbed through any mucous membrane, and is carried by the blood to the heart, lungs, and the rest of the body. Taken intranasally, it reaches the brain and neurons of the central nervous system in 3 minutes. It is metabolized rapidly by the blood and liver. Its actions on the sympathetic nervous system mimic the body's "fight-or-flight" response to fear or challenge, the same way an extremely stressful situation would. Cocaine is a vasoconstrictor, narrowing the blood vessels. It accelerates heart rate, blood pressure, and respiration, along with the overall metabolism of the body. Appetite and the need for sleep are suppressed. Its physical action is almost identical to that of amphetamines, except that the latter's actions are longer-lasting. Inhaled, the drug's effects peak in 15-20 minutes, and usually disappear in 60-90 minutes, although some people continue to suffer from adverse and even life-threatening effects for several hours after drug use has ceased.

Cocaine stimulates at least two areas of the brain—the cerebral cortex (which governs functions such as memory and reasoning) and the hypothalamus (which is responsible for appetite, body temperature, sleep, and certain emotional reactions). The extreme euphoria associated with cocaine use resembles that produced by direct electrical stimulation of the reward centers of the brain. Research done at Fair Oaks Hospital in Summit, New Jersey, shows that repeated use of the drug upsets the delicate balance of three neurotransmitters—norepinephrine, epinephrine, and dopamine, with special effects on the latter. These chemical messengers have a natural stimulant effect on the brain. Cocaine causes brain cells to release their supplies of all three, and blocks their re-uptake by the brain, eventually causing an exhaustion of the natural supply (see Figures 4 and 5 on page 122. After constant use, the brain craves this stimulation, leading to the mental agonies of cocaine withdrawal. Disruption of the dopamine processes is now thought to be responsible for some of the symptoms of cocaine-induced psychosis. This devastating effect is thought to be reversible after all cocaine use has ceased.

METHOD OF ABUSE

Cocaine hydrochloride is "snorted" (inhaled) through the nose. A small quantity of the powder is placed on a mirror or smooth stone surface, chopped with a razor blade to remove flakes and lumps, and formed into "lines" that are normally about 1 to 2 inches long and 1/8-inch wide. The cocaine is then inhaled through a straw, store-bought cocaine snorter, or rolled-up currency.

The cocaine inhaled is "cut" (diluted) four to eight times with various substances. Some, like the sugars mannitol, lactose, and sucrose, merely add volume. Others are less expensive stimulants, such as caffeine, phenylpropanolamine, ephedrine, and amphetamine. The coke can also be cut with local anesthetics, such as procaine, lidocaine, and benzocaine. (In fact, before being classified as a narcotic under the Harrison Narcotic Act of 1914, many people used the drug for its anesthetic effects. Today, cocaine's medical applications are limited to use as a highly diluted anesthetic by ear, nose, and throat specialists, proctologists, and cosmetic surgeons.)

BEHAVIORAL AND PSYCHOLOGICAL EFFECTS

Cocaine causes mood elevation; absence of depression and fatigue; lack of inhibition; feelings of power, increased intelligence, and self-confidence; insomnia; appetite suppression; nervousness; hyperexcitability; and excesses in speech and movement. Users may try to solve problems such as shyness, obesity, fatigue, and depression with cocaine. Some people experience heightened self-awareness; altered sexual feelings (which are at first enhanced, but then with repeated use decrease to the point of impotence or frigidity); a diminished sense of humor; less involvement with the real world and the needs of others; perceptual changes such as distortion, mild hallucination, misjudgment of size and distance, and a feeling of flying; and compulsive behavior (repeating the same task over and over again without realizing it, or constant grinding of the teeth).

Once the initial cocaine "rush" wears off, the down side appears, and becomes increasingly pronounced with constant use. In this stage, the user feels depressed, extremely anxious (to the degree of having severe "panic attacks"), irritable, hostile, alienated, fearful, confused, and paranoid. The more the drug is used, the more noticeable these symptoms become. In extreme cases, users may experience a temporary but complete split with reality—known as cocaine psychosis. Symptoms of this reaction often mimic schizophrenia and extreme paranoia. The user can become violent, and may experience visual, auditory, or tactile hallucinations (the most common of which is the sensation of insects crawling under the skin). Cocaine psychosis can last from a few days to a few months and requires immediate hospitalization.

PHYSICAL EFFECTS

The effects of cocaine on the body are all profound and adverse. They include: rapid pulse rate; elevated blood pressure; increased breathing rate; high body temperature; headache; sweating; dilated eye pupils; abdominal pain; nausea; vomiting; elevated blood sugar levels; vitamin, mineral and amino-acid deficiency with repeated use; the urge to defecate or urinate constantly; belching; dry mouth; the tightening of muscles (including those controlling bowel movements); loss of appetite; and slowed digestion.

Most patients in cocaine treatment centers show deficiencies in at least one vitamin—usually vitamin B1, B6, or C—due to poor and erratic eating habits. They also suffer from chronic runny noses, nosebleeds, sores, upper respiratory infections, inflammations of the liver (hepatitis), and sometimes of the heart lining (endocarditis). Most cocaine users appear to have the symptoms of a head cold, such as sneezing and congestion. Chronic cocaine abusers may eventually suffer from septal necrosis—the destruction of the mucous membranes and cartilage that separate the two nostrils. This condition must be repaired surgically.

Effects on the respiratory system also include inflammation of the trachea and bronchii, hoarseness or complete loss of the voice (more common in cocaine smokers), and chronic heavy coughing. Damage to the cardiovascular system includes irregular heart contractions, extremely rapid heart rate, increased blood pressure to the point where hemorrhage or congestive heart failure can result, chest pain from blood vessels around the heart (angina pectoris), and heart attack.

There are special health conditions that cocaine use can aggravate. It can cause or exacerbate bronchitis and upper respiratory infections; trigger asthma attacks in vulnerable people; magnify generalized anxiety to the point where hospitalization is needed; intensify depression to suicidal levels; aggravate circulatory problems because it constricts blood vessels; trigger heart attacks and/or increase existing heart problems; bring on seizures in epileptics; and endanger the lives of diabetics, because the drug increases blood sugar levels. A cocaine user's poor diet, lack of sleep, and ravaged metabolism also reduces immunity to all types of infections.

EFFECTS ON PREGNANCY

Experiments done with animals suggest that cocaine use by a pregnant woman may lead to eye and bone defects in her unborn child. The drug appears to constrict the blood vessels of the placenta, reducing the supply of blood (and therefore oxygen and nutrients) reaching the fetus. Cocaine use is also thought to contribute to the separation of the placenta from the wall of the uterus, premature birth, and stillbirth. There is a greater tendency to miscarry, and some doctors now believe this is due to strokes being suffered by the fetus itself. Babies born to cocaine-using women are often irritable and jittery in their first days of life. The drug can also be transferred from a woman to her infant through breast milk. In addition, women who chronically use cocaine tend to be malnourished, which can cause a wide range of birth defects, and lead to nutrient deficiencies in the child who is breast-fed.

DOSAGES

The amount of cocaine hydrochloride a person uses varies considerably. One "line" of cocaine averages about 25 milligrams, 60 percent of which is absorbed through the mucuous membranes of the body. Some casual users may snort only 100 milligrams daily; chronic users on "binges"— where cocaine is continuously used until the money or the user is exhausted—can take as many as 5 grams or more. However, while users develop a tolerance to the cocaine "high," they do not develop the same tolerance to the drug's cardiovascular actions.

In 1977 the American Medical Association suggested that the maximum safe dose of cocaine, when clinically administered, is 200 milligrams per 70 kilograms (155 pounds) of body weight, or 3.5 milligrams per kilogram (2.2 pounds) of weight, every 30 minutes. But death and/or cocaine psychosis can occur in some people even at these levels, and at lower levels still when street cocaine, cut with substances the user may be specifically sensitive to, is involved. Some people are cocaine-sensitive, and even a relatively tiny amount can result in overdose and possibly death. Experts agree that a single fatal dose of pure cocaine is somewhere between 1.2 and 1.4 grams taken orally by a person weighing 150 pounds.

TOXIC EFFECTS AND OVERDOSE

In addition to heart and lung damage, along with cocaine psychosis, users can suffer from other extreme toxic reactions. Chronic users sometimes report a phenomenon known as "snow lights," which are flashes of light in the periphery of vision. Eye specialists have detected small crystals in the retinas of some of these individuals. Intravenous users risk hepatitis, AIDS, and other infections from contaminated needles.

The most common causes of death from cocaine abuse are respiratory paralysis, heart rhythm disturbances, and repeated convulsions, usually from massive doses at the end of a binge. Also, some users die due to allergic reactions to the adulterants ("cuts").

Death from a cocaine overdose is quick: a user with no previous symptoms lapses suddenly into grand mal convulsions, followed in about 1 minute by respiratory collapse and death. Sudden death is infrequent and appears to be unpredictable, affecting those who may have used as little as 60 milligrams. Some researchers suggest that this is due to the fact that certain people lack an enzyme that destroys circulating cocaine.

Users may also die from highway or industrial accidents caused by lack of judgment, from suicide, or in the case of serious use and dealing, from murder, which is not uncommon in the cocaine-selling community.

TOLERANCE, ADDICTION, AND WITHDRAWAL

Previously, some experts felt that users did not develop a true physical addiction to cocaine. But recent evidence shows that the dopamine-starved brain does crave cocaine after withdrawal. So all the necessary requirements for physical and psychological dependence are present:

compulsive use, increasing tolerance, and withdrawal symptoms.

Classic withdrawal symptoms associated with narcotic addiction, such as delirium, muscle cramps, and convulsions, are not present when cocaine use is terminated. But chronic abusers do suffer from brain-wave and sleep-pattern changes, agitation, deep depression, anxiety, sleep disturbances, irritability, and an intense craving for cocaine. Withdrawing patients may have bouts of extreme hunger broken up by long periods of sleep. They complain of dreams and nightmares concerning cocaine use, and severe feelings of inferiority. People who have used cocaine in large amounts for a long period of time suffer from the most extreme withdrawal symptoms and are prone to relapse in the first month or two of outpatient treatment. That is why hospitalization is recommended for those with serious, long-term addictions.

OPTIONS FOR TREATMENT

There is no definitive or best treatment for cocaine abuse. The form of care depends on the person, and the extent of the problem. Treatment can range from the cautious use of drugs to control the depression and anxiety brought on by cocaine withdrawal, to simply providing quiet surroundings and self-help groups while the individual recovers. If the person has strong personal resources—a good job, good self-esteem, drug-free friends and family who are willing to support his efforts— outpatient treatment is often the best route. However, if these things are missing, and if the patient's immediate environment is filled with drug-using peers, then hospitalization is advised, and could last from a few weeks to a year.

Some doctors use medication at the start of treatment. Sedatives such as diazepam (Valium) are prescribed for cocaine-induced anxiety, and if the patient is suffering from psychotic symptoms, a stronger drug may be temporarily added, such as a phenothiazine-derivative antipsychotic agent. Because cocaine use sometimes masks underlying depression, people with this problem may be given an antidepressant medication. The Fair Oaks Hospital in Summit, New Jersey, uses tyrosine (used by the brain to make dopamine and norepinephrine) in battling such withdrawal effects as fearfulness, insomnia, trembling, and nausea. A dopamine substitute, bromocriptine, has shown initial promise in studies for reducing post-use symptoms and cravings in hospitalized patients. But there can be no pharmaceutical substitutes for the behavioral, psychological, and lifestyle changes needed for recovery from any chemical dependency.

The first thing a person who has decided to stop using the drug should do is see his doctor. This will determine whether or not cocaine use has seriously damaged the body, whether nutritional deficiencies exist, and whether drug use has been masking some previously existing condition. The doctor can refer the patient to a drug treatment program, or the patient can contact state agencies for a referral. Inpatient programs include hospital drug treatment units and therapeutic communities, where residents work together to cook meals, tend the grounds, etc.

People with strong personal resources can explore an outpatient program, where drug education and counseling are offered several times a week. Treatment in such centers often involves a contract with the patient for an initial 30-day abstinence period (verified by constant urine testing), with the stipulation that the patient will be hospitalized immediately if drug use starts again.

Psychological counseling should deal with present problems and strategies for the future, rather than using in-depth psychoanalysis. Family members should be encouraged to participate in group sessions. Self-help groups on the order of Alcoholics Anonymous (such as Cocaine Anonymous) are also necessary.

In recent years, acupuncture treatment has given considerable relief to cocaine abusers. (Its ability to control withdrawal may be due to neurochemical activity and the possibility that the procedure stimulates the production of natural endorphins—the brain-produced chemicals often called the body's own morphine.)

Behavior modification programs, using relaxation techniques and hypnosis, are used to try to change patterns of behavior that led to drug use. The patient must break all ties with drug-using associates and find new activities and interests to replace drug use, or severe depression and/or relapse can occur.

Exercise is also advised, and the avoidance of all types of drugs (including alcohol) must be part of a lifelong program.

Contingency contracting is a new technique that takes the form of self-blackmail to keep patients in outpatient treatment. Upon entering a program to cure cocaine abuse, users "contract" to stick to the treatment and stay clear of the drug for a set period of time (usually 3 months). Should they violate that contract, the clinic will mail out letters written by the user at the time the contract was signed. These letters contain confessions of drug abuse, and can be addressed to employers, licensing boards, newspapers, relatives, or wherever they would cause the person serious trouble. These letters may also contain contributions to causes the user detests. A one-year test of the program at two clinics operated by the University of Colorado School of Medicine found that over 80 percent of contract-signing users made it through the 3-month period, while none of the users without a contract stayed drug-free for more than 4 weeks.

In choosing a program, families should visit with staff members, check references and the history of the program, ask questions about insurance coverage, length of stay that will be covered, and any hidden costs.

(See Chapter Twenty-Four for a detailed discussion of chemical dependency treatment programs, as well as a list of numbers to call for help.)

LONG-TERM PROGNOSIS

Cocaine addiction is one of the most difficult forms of chemical dependency to overcome, particularly if the patient lacks support from family and friends, and does not have a good education or solid employment. While there are no hard and fast figures to indicate how many people recover from cocaine dependency, it is generally thought that people who functioned well before their trouble with drugs will function well again once they rid their lives of drug dependency. Motivation and sincerity are vital in starting treatment. Most drug users initially deny they have a problem, but once they come to terms with it, they have a much greater chance of success.

Cocaine users may lose their money, employment and families in the course of addiction. They also may be left with chronic heart and respiratory problems, as well as digestive ailments. Some compound the problem by abusing other drugs, such as alcohol, marijuana, depressants, or opiates, along with cocaine use. These people are harder to treat, and their attempts to stay off drugs may be a lifelong struggle.

CRACK (FREEBASE SMOKING)

METHOD OF ACTION

Smoking crack and freebasing have the same effects on body and mind and are essentially the same activity. The only difference is in the way the cocaine is prepared for smoking. Crack also generally contains more impurities from the "cuts" used in the original cocaine hydrochloride. When cocaine is smoked, greater amounts of cocaine reach the brain and sympathetic nervous system with incredible speed—about 7 seconds. This produces a more intense "high," a more devastating "down," and a much quicker route to tolerance and addiction.

METHOD OF ABUSE

Crack, which is sold in a ready-to-use form in small vials containing a few slivers or rocks, is smoked either in a pipe with water, a corn-cob pipe, or in a cigarette containing marijuana or tobacco.

Freebase (the purified base form of cocaine processed from the hydrochloride salt using volatile chemicals such as ether) is typically smoked through a water pipe. The average "hit" off the pipe involves about 120 milligrams of cocaine. The apex of the rush is achieved in approximately 90 seconds, and the effects dissipate into depression, cravings, and nervousness within a few minutes.

Another way cocaine is smoked is by placing a small amount of freebase or crack on a piece of foil, which is heated from below by a match or lighter. The rising wisps of smoke are inhaled. This process is known as "chasing the dragon," particularly when it is done with heroin.

Coca paste, the first extraction of the manufacturing process, can also be smoked in a cigarette, but this method is not popular yet in this country.

BEHAVIORAL AND PSYCHOLOGICAL EFFECTS

The effects of smoking cocaine are much like the effects of snorting it—except more powerful, quicker, and more dangerous. Cocaine psychosis, hallucinations, and delusions of paranoia are not uncommon among crack smokers, and violence is another unpleasant by-product. Crack smoking can lead to addiction in less than 2 months, whereas it normally takes years for a person snorting cocaine to become as dependent on the drug.

The "high" a user gets from smoking cocaine is immediate and intense. Feelings of power, intellect, and self-confidence are extreme. So is the depletion of neurotransmitters in the brain. The high is very short-lived: it is gone in a matter of minutes, and the user must smoke again to dispel the unpleasant feelings of the crash. For this reason, crack smokers routinely go on "binges"—they consume vast quantities of the drug in a 24-hour period, until their money or strength runs out. These binges may take place where the drug is sold, in residences called "crack houses." Crack, unlike cocaine, is not normally used at social occasions such as rock concerts or dinner parties. The rush is so intense people want to use it quietly and in private. A normal social and professional life soon disappears.

Crack users say that coming down from a hit of the drug occurs in five stages:

1. Worry about where the user can get more crack
2. Deep depression and intense anxiety
3. Loss of energy and appetite
4. Insomnia
5. Intense love/hate feelings for self

The rush from smoking cocaine is so intense and the crash so powerful, users are focused on nothing but the next hit of the drug. Addicts will resort to robbery, prostitution, and even murder to obtain more. Attention to diet, sleep, or personal cleanliness ceases. Freebase smokers often abuse other drugs, such as opiates, in order to ease the pain of coming down.

Freebase smoking can lead to radical changes in behavior and personality, including extreme depression, irritability, hostility, social withdrawal, paranoia, and violent and/or suicidal behavior. Although no one is completely sure about the long-term effects of crack abuse, many experts believe that these changes may be permanent if enough crack is smoked for a long period of time.

PHYSICAL EFFECTS

The effects of crack and freebase are those of cocaine—intensified. Immediate symptoms are a chronic sore throat and hoarseness, gasping for breath, and a hacking cough that produces black phlegm. Cocaine smokers become extremely vulnerable to emphysema and other severe respiratory problems and infections. Users are said to lose weight, develop skin problems, and suffer from convulsions. Crack (and cocaine) slows digestion and hunger; creates euphoria, agitation, restlessness, and apprehensiveness; stimulates the central nervous system; elevates blood pressure, temperature, pulse, blood sugar, and thirst; promotes sexual arousal at first but then causes complete loss of interest in sex; and can cause cardiovascular problems and death. The "cuts" used in the original cocaine can also affect heart rhythm, blood pressure, and cause other general health problems when the cocaine is smoked, since these adulterants survive the extraction process in significant amounts and can get into the bloodstream through this method in fairly high doses.

Long-term use of crack can lead to serious heart ailments, severe digestive disorders (due to erratic eating habits and malnutrition), an extreme form of dehydration, anorexia, lowered resistance to disease, and even death by malnutrition.

EFFECTS ON PREGNANCY

Cocaine smoking carries with it the same kind of risks to mother and child that cocaine snorting does, only adverse effects are more intense and more common. Recent studies show preliminary evidence that babies born to crack-using mothers may develop learning disabilities and have a poor attention span. Future research will determine whether babies born to cocaine smokers or who drink the milk of such women may be suffering from permanent brain damage.

DOSAGES

Crack is preprocessed and sold in vials that contain several small chunks. The vials now come in at least five sizes, from .3cc to .85cc and sell from $5 to $450. The sizes most frequently sold are $10 and $20 vials. Dealers profit tremendously from selling crack because it "hooks" clients so quickly. Although initially it appears cheaper because it is sold in smaller quantities, it costs as much ($100 a gram) as cocaine powder. It ends up costing the user more money than the powder form, because crack is used more quickly. Freebase smokers have been known to consume 30 grams in a 24-hour period. Because each "hit" of smoke can contain 67-120 milligrams of cocaine in concentrated form, any amount of freebase use carries the risk of overdose.

TOXIC EFFECTS AND OVERDOSE

The extremely high blood levels of cocaine produced by freebase smoking increase the likelihood of serious toxic reactions, including potentially fatal brain seizures, irregular heartbeat, complete cardiac and respiratory arrest resulting in sudden death, and critically high blood pressure that can lead to strokes. Lung and heart damage can be permanent.

Serious respiratory problems in chronic smokers include chest congestion, wheezing, black phlegm, chronic cough, and general impairment of lung function. Other problems include hoarseness to the point of voice loss, parched lips, tongue and throat, and singed eyebrows and eyelashes.

Cocaine-induced psychosis, previously described, can last for several months. In a case where the user has a pre-existing mental problem, it can last for life.

Industrial, household, and car accidents are common among crack users, as well as suicide, murder, and death by drowning (many users swim to relieve the parched feeling).

Freebase smoking involving the use of volatile chemicals can lead to explosions and burns. "Formication," the sensation of insects crawling under the skin, has been reported in many cocaine smokers. Some users have torn holes in their bodies trying to remove the "bugs." Other forms of hallucinations and delusions are also common. Both cocaine-induced brain seizures and cocaine-induced psychosis are more likely to affect adolescents than adults, but no heavy cocaine user is immune.

TOLERANCE, ADDICTION, AND WITHDRAWAL

Tolerance to cocaine smoking builds quickly within weeks, and addiction can occur anywhere from 6 to 10 weeks after initial exposure. While some casual users of cocaine hydrochloride may snort a line or two at a party but seldom buy or seriously abuse the drug, most repeat cocaine smokers become addicted.

Again, withdrawal from crack is the same as withdrawal from regular cocaine use, but highly intensified. The crack or freebase user is more likely to need hospitalization because of serious medical and psychiatric problems and extremely intense cravings.

OPTIONS FOR TREATMENT

Most crack abusers must be treated initially in a hospital setting, first to determine the extent of physical and psychological damage, and second, to keep the patient away from the drug during the period of most intense craving. Therapeutic communities are often recommended. Crack users should be checked for heart and lung damage, as well as malnutrition. They should then be sent for evaluation and treatment to a substance abuse program that offers cocaine-specific treatment, and has both in-patient and outpatient services. The person with strong resources (high motivation, good job, supportive family) may try an outpatient program first, but only when use has not been chronic and profound.

The physician may choose to use sedatives or neurotransmitter-replacing drugs to lessen the symptoms of withdrawal, or may have to prescribe an antipsychotic agent if more profound psychological disturbances appear. The aim of any treatment program is to get the patient off all types of drugs, including alcohol, on a permanent basis.

Self-help programs (Cocaine Anonymous), group therapy, and individual counseling should be considered once the dependency has been treated.

LONG-TERM PROGNOSIS

Because cocaine-smoking is a relatively new phenomenon in the U.S. (freebasing appeared in the 1970s, crack in the early 1980s), there are few statistics to indicate how successful the treatment of dependent users has been. Experts do mention that crack users may be more likely to become permanently disabled for a number of reasons. First, unlike many abusers of cocaine powder, crack smokers are often from inner-city neighborhoods, from poorer socioeconomic environments, and so have fewer personal resources. Their friends and family members may also abuse drugs.

Second, the use of crack often leads to severe abuse of alcohol and other drugs. Depressants such as barbiturates and tranquilizers are taken to relieve the insomnia, anxiety, and restlessness. Heavy marijuana smoking is common, and some users take heroin or other opiates to counteract the side effects of "crashing." This results in multiple drug dependencies, which are always harder to treat successfully.

Third, and most unfortunately, chronic cocaine smoking can cause permanent heart, lung, liver, and psychological damage, making it harder for the ex-abuser to regain a normal lifestyle after treatment.

CHAPTER SIXTEEN

STIMULANTS:
Amphetamines

GENERIC AND BRAND NAMES

Amphetamines

amphetamine sulfate *(Benzedrine)*

dextroamphetamine sulfate *(Dexedrine)*

amphetamine with dextroamphetamine *(Biphetamine)*

methamphetamine hydrochloride *(Desoxyn, Methedrine)*

Non-amphetamines with a similar chemical action

phenmetrazine hydrochloride *(Preludin)*

methylphenidate hydrochloride *(Ritalin)* (also see Chapter Eleven)

pemoline *(Cylert)* (also see Chapter Eleven)

Anorectic drugs

benzphetamine *(Didrex)*

chlorphentermine *(Pre-Sate)*

chlortermine *(Voranil)*

diethylpropion *(Tenuate, Tepanil)*

fenfluramine *(Pondimin)*

mazindol *(Sanorex, Mazanor)*

phendimetrazine *(Plegine, Bacarate, Melfiat, Statobex, Tanorex)*

phentermine *(Ionamin, Adipex-P)*

In America, many people believe that to be successful they must move faster, look thinner, and work harder. This may have led to a society-wide interest in stimulant drugs, the most popular of which at this time is cocaine. Prior to cocaine's popularity, the other class of stimulants—drugs loosely known as "speed"—were abused more regularly among all classes of society. Amphetamine and amphetamine-like compounds were used to cure fatigue, to sharpen the senses and mind, to lose weight, or to work harder and longer hours, not to mention just to "get high." In the past, many of these drugs were legally prescribed and monitored—the problems appeared when people abused them or obtained them illegally. Today these drugs are rarely prescribed except in special cases, such as for temporary weight loss or the treatment of hyperactivity in children, and most people who abuse them obtain them through illicit means.

These psychoactive drugs, with their rapid tolerance and addiction levels, can cause devastating physical and psychological effects on chronic users. Although amphetamine use has decreased in recent years—and doctors are very cautious in prescribing such drugs—there is still a large problem due mostly to bootleg manufacturers. Legal production of these substances, which peaked in 1971 when over 12 billion "diet pills" were produced, declined to the point that by 1980, only 2 million amphetamine prescriptions were processed in the nation's pharmacies.

A large number of people use some form of stimulant during the day—nicotine and caffeine being the most common. While these drugs are associated with many health risks, more potent stimulants can be more dangerous. Users tend to rely on them to feel stronger, more decisive, and self-confident. However, due to the cumulative effects of the drugs, chronic abusers often follow a pattern of taking "uppers" in the morning and "downers" such as alcohol or sleeping pills at night. Such chemical manipulation interferes with normal body processes and can lead to mental and physical illness. Young people who use stimulants for their euphoric effects may consume large doses sporadically, often over weekends or at night, and may eventually begin experimenting with other drugs of abuse.

The long-term use of stimulants is followed by a period of discomfort known as "crashing," with symptoms such as anxiety, restlessness, and depression. The only way to counteract these effects is to take more and more of the drugs.

Amphetamine, dextroamphetamine, and methamphetamine are very similar in their effects, differing only in degrees. Amphetamine is a synthetically produced stimulant, developed in Germany during the 1880s. At first, as with heroin, it was considered safe and was widely prescribed to treat everything from asthma to narcolepsy (a rare disorder resulting in the uncontrollable tendency to fall asleep). Benzedrine inhalers for asthma patients became popular in the 1930s. When amphetamines came into widespread use, either in prescription form or in over-the-counter inhalers and preparations, their abuse spread to many groups, from housewives to students to truck drivers. Their effect as appetite suppressants made them a highly popular way to lose weight.

Those addicted to the drugs, often called "speed freaks," became known for their bizarre and sometimes violent behavior, as well as for the vast quantities of the drugs they would consume. Whereas a prescribed dose is between 2.5 and 15 milligrams per day, those on a speed binge might inject as much as 100 milligrams every two to three hours. The recognition of the harmful effects of amphetamine use and its limited therapeutic value led to tighter controls and far fewer prescriptions. The compounds were taken out of over-the-counter products. The medical use of amphetamines is now limited to narcolepsy, attention deficit disorders in children (see Chapter Eleven), and certain cases of obesity (as a short-term adjunct to a restricted diet for patients who do not respond to other forms of therapy). But underground laboratories produce vast quantities of amphetamines, particularly methamphetamine, for distribution on the illicit market.

The most hyper-charged of all the different forms of speed is called *crystal*, the street name for methamphetamine. It is sold in powdered form and can be injected, inhaled, or taken orally. It produces an intense wave of physical and psychological exhilaration upon injection or absorption, along with a rapid deterioration of physical and psychological health following extended use. There are very few old crystal abusers on the street.

Crank is the recognized name for street speed, especially of the pill variety. This term covers pharmaceutical and bootleg amphetamines. For the most part the objective and subjective effects are the same as those produced by crystal, only to a lesser degree.

Lookalikes are tablets and capsules made to simulate prescription amphetamines but which contain only legally available non-prescription stimulants, decongestants, and antihistamines. They emerged in the late 1970s as a result of the increasing scarcity of amphetamines on the street. The ingredients are usually blends of caffeine, ephedrine, and phenylpropanolamine, compounds which are in a number of over-the-counter stimulants and diet aids. These "innocent" ingredients can have devastating side effects, however, especially in people who have a marked sensitivity to them. Deaths have been triggered by massive sudden increases in blood pressure produced by these drugs. The blood pressure can become so high in hypersensitive users that cerebral hemorrhage results.

Hallucinogenic amphetamines, such as MDA, are amphetamine-based psychedelics that may be injected, snorted, or ingested, and have similar effects to other hallucinogens. They will be discussed in further detail in Chapter Nineteen.

The medical indications, patterns of abuse, and adverse effects of *non-amphetamine stimulants* such as phenmetrazine (Preludin) and methylphenidate (Ritalin) compare closely with those of other stimulants. Phenmetrazine is medically used only as an appetite suppressant, and methylphenidate is used mainly for the treatment of attention-deficit disorders in children. While the abuse of these drugs involves both oral and intravenous use, most users inject tablets that have been dissolved in water. Complications arising from this practice are common because the tablets contain insoluble materials that, upon injection, block small blood vessels and cause serious damage, especially in the lungs and retina of the eye.

In recent years a number of medications, called *anorectic drugs*, have been manufactured and marketed to replace amphetamines as appetite suppressants. They produce many of the effects of amphetamines but are generally less potent. All are controlled because of the similarity of their effects to those of other stimulants. Fenfluramine differs somewhat from the others because at low doses it produces sedation. Pemoline (Cylert) is now a commonly used drug for the treatment of attention-deficit disorders in children.

During the 1960s, when amphetamine use was booming, people began wearing a button that summarizes the experience of those who chronically abused these drugs. The button's message was clear and simple. It read, "Speed Kills."

METHOD OF ACTION

These drugs are well-absorbed from the digestive tract, especially in the case of dextroamphetamine and methamphetamine. They cause clinical effects within 30 minutes after oral ingestion. Depending on the strength of the drug, subjective and objective reactions can last from several hours to a few days. The stimulation of the central nervous system, the anorexia, and the psychomotor activity probably result from the increased release of norepinephrine and dopamine from nerve endings in the brain, or by interference with the normal breakdown of these released neurotransmitters, leading to chronically increased levels in the brain. The paranoid psychosis that sometimes accompanies long-term use may result from the effects of high dopamine levels.

METHOD OF ABUSE

Speed is either taken orally in tablets or capsules, snorted as a powder, or injected from powder or crushed tablet form. Injection carries with it many health risks because of insoluble materials in the crushed tablets, or because of AIDS caused by using shared needles. The powder may burn intensely when snorted.

BEHAVIORAL AND PSYCHOLOGICAL EFFECTS

While taking low to moderate doses, users may experience: increased alertness, wakefulness, elevation of mood, mild euphoria, increased athletic performance, decreased fatigue, an absence of boredom, less mental clouding with resulting clearer thinking, improved concentration, increased energy, increased irritability, restlessness, insomnia, blurred vision, and anxiety.

At high doses, a drug-induced psychosis may result, causing confused and disorganized behavior, the compulsive repetition of meaningless acts, irritability, fear, paranoia, hallucinations, and delusions. The user may become aggressive and extremely antisocial, even to the point of violence. The attitude of many chronic amphetamine abusers may mimic that of a manic depressive in the manic stage, with grandiose gestures and beliefs about oneself, excessive spending, unrealistic goals, etc. Driving a car or operating machinery while using these drugs is ill-advised, because of altered judgment or excessive belief in one's own abilities.

PHYSICAL EFFECTS

Possible physical effects of stimulant abuse include increased blood pressure, cardiac palpitations, disturbed digestion, anorexia, nausea, headaches, sweating, dry mouth, skin sores, malnutrition, infections resulting from neglected health care, an increase in body temperature, sleep disturbances, and slowed heart rate. Damage to organs, particularly the lungs, liver, and kidneys, can also easily result from long-term use. Other physical side effects include increased blood sugar, increased blood flow to the muscles, decreased blood flow to the organs, dilated pupils, increased respiration, and slight tremors. Prolonged episodes of intoxication from methamphetamine ("speed runs") are accompanied by anorexia, weight loss, insomnia, and generalized deterioration in psychomotor abilities. Injected methamphetamine in large doses may cause chest pain, temporary paralysis, or the inability to function.

EFFECTS ON PREGNANCY

Amphetamine use by pregnant women increases the chances of miscarriage and may cause heart defects and cleft palates in newborns. Babies of heavy amphetamine abusers may be agitated and then depressed right after birth. These drugs can also affect the later development of the babies and contribute to a lack of coordination and poor responsiveness to their surroundings.

DOSAGES

Dose ranges are different for all amphetamines. In general, low to moderate doses are 5-50 milligrams orally, and high doses are 100 milligrams intravenously. Dextroamphetamine is more potent than simple amphetamine, and so low to moderate doses are 2.5 to 20 milligrams and high doses are 50 milligrams. Chronic use of over 100 milligrams in any form can lead to toxic psychosis with its schizophrenia-like symptoms. Tolerance to the toxic effects of amphetamines and methamphetamines varies. Some patients become ill taking 30 milligrams, while other chronic users can tolerate one gram or more of dextroamphetamine. Methamphetamine abusers on a "speed run" may take in large doses every few hours.

TOXIC EFFECTS AND OVERDOSE

People suffering from acute intoxication may show restlessness, irritability, tremor, confusion, talkativeness, anxiety, and a changeable mood. They may suffer from headache, chills, vomiting, dry mouth, sweating, an irregular heartbeat, and changes in blood pressure. In severe cases, auditory and visual hallucinations, toxic psychosis, seizures, and increased body temperatures result. Chronic infections, malnutrition, and damage to body organs can accompany long-term abuse.

The toxic psychosis that occurs with abuse of these drugs appears with symptoms such as: fear; increased aggression; delusions of persecution; auditory, visual and tactile hallucinations; grinding or gnashing of the teeth; a distorted sense of time; changes in the perception of the body image; hyperactivity; and compulsive behavior (characterized by the doing and undoing of a particular task).

Death from amphetamine overdose is not common but far from impossible. In the absence of medical intervention, high fever, convulsions, and cardiovascular collapse may precede death. Physical exertion increases the hazards of stimulant use, since accidental death is due in part to the effects on the cardiovascular and temperature-regulating systems. Fatalities following extreme exertion have been reported among athletes who have taken stimulants in moderate amounts.

TOLERANCE, ADDICTION, AND WITHDRAWAL

Tolerance develops rapidly to both the euphoric and appetite-suppressant effects. Doses large enough to overcome the insensitivity that develops can cause mental aberrations and physical illness. If withdrawn from stimulants, chronic high-dose users exhibit profound depression, apathy, fatigue, and disturbed sleep (increased REM sleep) for up to 20 hours a day.

The immediate withdrawal syndrome may last several days, but there can be lingering impairment of perception and thought processes. Anxiety, an incapacitating tenseness, and suicidal tendencies may persist for weeks or months. Many experts now interpret these symptoms as indicating that stimulant drugs cause physical dependence. Whether the withdrawal symptoms are physical or psychological is academic, because stimulants are recognized as among the most potent agents of reward and reinforcement that underlie the problem of dependence.

OPTIONS FOR TREATMENT

Amphetamine abusers should first check with a medical doctor to see if drug use has caused or masked any serious physical or psychological conditions. Treatment with medication for toxicity, toxic psychosis, or the symptoms of withdrawal may be required in a hospital setting. Seizures may be treated with diazepam (Valium), and ammonium chloride (to increase the rate of secretion of the drug). Psychotic symptoms may need chlorpromazine (Thorazine) or similar antipsychotic agents administered over several days.

Long-term treatment may consist of hospitalization in a residential program, especially in cases where depression and some psychotic symptoms persist after the initial withdrawal period. A structured outpatient program with several meetings per week is often successful for people with strong personal resources. Self-help groups and the support of family and friends can go a long way toward helping the patient recover.

However, apart from treating psychotic symptoms, the use of other drugs is not advised. While sedatives may help the patient sleep during the weeks after stimulant abuse is terminated, they offer no long-term solutions to insomnia. Antidepressants—even though they perk up a person's mood—provide real help only for amphetamine users whose depression has a biological basis.

LONG-TERM PROGNOSIS

With proper treatment and support, stimulant abusers have a good chance of recovering, especially if there are no accompanying dependencies on other drugs (i.e., barbiturates, alcohol). In most cases, victims of toxic psychosis exhibit a slow but complete recovery in a few days to a few weeks, unless there is an underlying psychiatric problem. However, psychotic symptoms have been known to persist for years. Sufferers have an amazingly accurate memory of these psychiatric episodes and can explain them in detail.

Long-term amphetamine abuse can take a more serious physical toll. The strain that these drugs place on the cardiovascular system can lead to several problems—hypertension, irregular heart rhythm and stroke. Injury to small blood vessels serving the eye can damage the retina. And brain damage is a possibility, particularly to users who inject the drug. Intravenous use can lead to infections, blood poisoning, hepatitis and AIDS. The heavy use of methamphetamine may cause small blood vessels serving the brain to deteriorate and rupture, resulting in permanent damage.

CHAPTER SEVENTEEN

CANNABINOIDS:
Marijuana and Hashish

Everyone is familiar with marijuana—the love and peace drug of the 1960s, the drug for "harmless" recreational fun. Few other psychoactive substances have inspired as much debate, engendered as much print, and ill-deserved such a good name. People have recommended legalizing it, claiming it is safer than alcohol. Although its use has decreased somewhat since its hippie heyday, it is estimated that 60 percent of all American high school seniors have tried it, and nearly one out of 14 is a daily user. Many first-time marijuana users are as young as 9 years old. The facts about this friendly drug are not so comforting, however. An ever-increasing bulk of evidence indicates that marijuana damages the brain, heart, lungs, and reproductive system.

Proponents of legalization point to the fact that marijuana appears to have some therapeutic uses: in the treatment of nausea resulting from chemotherapy, for reducing eyeball pressure in open-angle glaucoma, for epilepsy, and for people suffering from some form of muscle spasticity (as the result of conditions such as multiple sclerosis). The fact is that many of these therapeutic benefits have not yet been proven, and the substances contained within marijuana that have these positive effects may one day be duplicated with analogs (drugs similar in nature and structure to another drug) that would not be as harmful as marijuana itself.

Marijuana (cannabis) is one of the ancient folk medicines. Until 50 years ago, physicians occasionally used the plant to treat lockjaw, depression, toothache, constipation, and a variety of other disorders. To understand why it appears to have so many positive effects, one must remember that the drug has some sedative properties. Therefore, by possibly allaying the fears and anxieties associated with a multitude of illnesses, its use makes the patient feel better.

Cannabis has been known for both its narcotic qualities and its fiber for thousands of years. It is recorded in a Chinese herbal directory of 2737 B.C. It has been, and remains, widely used in many countries in Africa,

Asia, the Middle and Far East, and North and South America. The stem of the plant is also used in the manufacture of hemp rope and string.

Pharmacologically, it is a mild hallucinogen. It produces a lightheaded euphoria, but except in large doses, does not have the "trip" effect of stronger psychedelics such as LSD. Cannabis comes from a large plant, *Cannabis sativa*, which grows best in hot, dry climates. The whole plant, including the roots, is covered with small hairs, although the greatest concentration of them is on the flowering parts and top leaves. The hairs produce a sticky brown resin. The plants are dried and crumbled to produce marijuana, and the resin is collected and pressed into cakes known as hashish. There is also a liquid concentrate, commonly called hash oil.

To date, over 420 separate chemical entities have been isolated from the plant. Delta-9-tetrahydrocannabinol (better known as THC) is the major psychoactive component, although over 60 other cannabinoids are known. The potency of marijuana has increased dramatically since the 1960s, with more sophisticated growing techniques. In earlier years, confiscated marijuana rarely averaged above 0.5 percent THC, while more recent samples have shown levels from 4 percent to 10 percent THC. Hashish generally contains 20 percent; hash oil as much as 85 percent.

When marijuana is smoked, it produces more than 2000 different chemicals, the effects of which are not all known. The smoke also contains more tar, carbon monoxide, and known cancer-causing agents than does tobacco. The concentration of marijuana tar is 50-75 percent higher than in the same weight of tobacco tar. The amount of this carcinogen retained in the lungs from one marijuana cigarette ("joint") is probably even greater than from five normally smoked tobacco cigarettes, because cannabis smoke is inhaled deeply and held for as long as 30 seconds. Thus, two to three joints a day may carry the same risk of lung damage as smoking a pack of cigarettes.

Marijuana is by far the most frequently used and most easily obtained illicit substance. According to a 1982 Household Survey done by the Department of Justice, there are about 20 million annual users and about 4 million daily users, most of whom are adolescents and young adults. The effects on the young, who are in the early stages of both psychological and physiological development, are the most profound. Marijuana and hashish use is also part of what is known as the "gateway" phenomenon—the principle that the progression of drug use seems to go from beer or wine to cigarettes and hard liquor, to marijuana, and then to stronger illicit drugs, such as cocaine or heroin. Chronic marijuana users therefore may be more likely to graduate to more serious forms of drug abuse and dependency.

METHOD OF ACTION

Cannabis has stimulant, sedative, and hallucinogenic effects on the brain and body, which is why it is in a drug class of its own. Joints generally contain 0.5 to 1 gram of marijuana leaf with a THC content of 1-2 percent (5-20 milligrams). Absorption from lungs to bloodstream to brain varies, but the average experienced user will absorb approximately half the total dose into his bloodstream. Effects are felt almost immediately, and reach peak intensity within 30 minutes. The speed of onset is partially determined by the THC concentration.

After 1 hour, plasma levels decline and most subjective feelings disappear within 3 hours after the last dose. However, the fat solubility of THC, which is exceeded only by substances such as DDT, affects the way in which this substance is distributed within, and how long it remains in, the body. THC becomes concentrated in the fatty tissue and also lodges in the liver, lungs, reproductive organs, and the brain. The by-products of cannabis remain in body fat for several weeks with unknown consequences. It takes 3 days to a week for the body to rid itself of half the THC in a single joint, and up to 30 days to get rid of all of it. Some THC also remains bound to proteins in the blood.

There is strong evidence to indicate that cannabis produces acute effects on the brain, including chemical and electrophysiological changes. The areas and neurotransmitters in the brain concerned with learning and short-term memory appear to be the most severely affected.

METHOD OF ABUSE

The most common way of using cannabis is by smoking. A "joint" or "reefer" is a handmade cannabis cigarette, using the substance in place of, or with, tobacco, or mixing chips of hashish or hash oil with tobacco. These joints tend to be larger than conventional cigarettes, and may be rolled with two or three cigarette papers. Pipes, which come in all shapes and sizes, can also be used. To reduce the harshness of the smoke, the pipes may have a very long stem, or pass the smoke through water. A screen is usually put in the bowl of the pipe. If cannabis is smoked, its vapors are inhaled and held deeply within the lungs for at least several seconds before they are exhaled.

Cannabis can also be swallowed. It can be made into a tea or baked into cakes and other foods. If it is taken orally, it is 20-30 percent as effective, and the effects are experienced within 30-60 minutes. Subjective feelings persist for three to five hours, and the rate of absorption is affected by the food content of the stomach (the fuller the stomach, the slower the absorption).

People may smoke marijuana at the same time they are using cocaine or other stimulants, because of its mild sedative effects.

BEHAVIORAL AND PSYCHOLOGICAL EFFECTS

The effects of cannabis depend on the quantity and type consumed (some "brands" of marijuana and hashish are stronger than others) and on the user's mood, environment, and expectations. First-time users may not feel anything at all with low doses, or may experience a mild panic reaction with sensations of paranoia. For most people, it initially produces pleasurable feelings of mild euphoria and well-being—a type of lightheaded intoxication. Cannabis removes inhibitions, and the user may become excited, talkative, and relaxed. Larger doses can result in lethargy and confusion, with interference in many aspects of mental functioning (attention span, short-term memory, complex thought). Perception and motor coordination may be seriously affected, making driving or operating machinery hazardous. Large doses can result in intense feelings of paranoia or panic, aggressive or violent behavior (if the user is emotionally disturbed), depression, and even mild hallucinations and delusions. Confusion and disorientation are common. Sleepiness, increased appetite, occasional dizziness, increased auditory, visual and tactile perception, and relief from anxiety are all frequent effects of cannabis use.

Because with low doses marijuana's behavioral effects are not profound, people observing a user may not know he or she has taken the drug. But with high doses, toxic psychosis with hallucinations, panic, and delusions is possible, and the user's behavior will be severely altered.

Some people believe they can become more "creative" with marijuana use. While it has been shown in some studies that the drug changes thinking from left to right brain dominance, because of the mental confusion involved, creative endeavors appear to suffer from rather than be enhanced by cannabis abuse.

Acute intoxication interferes with mental functioning. Learning ability during marijuana or hashish abuse—both while the drug is smoked and during the period up to 30 days before the drug completely leaves the body—is diminished because of perceptual and memory difficulties. In addition, motivation and cognition may be altered, causing a decreased ability to process new information. The known and/or suspected chronic effects are short-term memory impairment and slowness of learning.

Marijuana also compromises all types of motor coordination and affects tracking ability and sensory and perceptual functions. It impairs driving skills for at least 4-6 hours after smoking a single joint. The use of marijuana in combination with alcohol causes a reduction in reaction time, poor cognition, and severely disturbed coordination.

There is increasing concern about the long-term developmental effects of marijuana use by children and adolescents. Clinicians use the term "amotivational syndrome" to describe behavioral and psychological changes that include: a pattern of energy loss, apathy, emotional blunting, loss of motivation or ambition, loss of effectiveness, hostility toward authority and discipline, disturbed parental and social relationships, diminished ability to carry out long-term plans, difficulty in concentrating, and a decline in school or work performance. Surveys have shown that 40 percent of heavy users experience some or all of these symptoms.

Heavy, chronic users also tend to lose interest in other types of pleasurable experiences, such as sex, outside hobbies, or recreational exercise.

PHYSICAL EFFECTS

The two most regularly observed physiologic effects are a substantial increase in heart rate and a dilation of the conjunctival vessels (red eye). Other physiological changes sometimes encountered include dry mouth, diarrhea, and drowsiness. However, the results of chronic use are profound and disturbing, and many experts believe that it affects most of the major systems of the body in the following ways:

• *Respiratory System Effects:* Runny nose (rhinitis), sore throat, bronchitis, chronic cough, the possibility of lung function impairment and cancer of the respiratory tract. Precancerous changes not normally seen in heavy tobacco smokers under the age of 40 have been found in small samples of bronchial tissue from 20-year-old heavy smokers of hashish with tobacco.

• *Cardiovascular System Effects:* Acceleration of heart beat and increased blood pressure in certain susceptible people. These changes pose a threat for people with abnormal heart and circulatory conditions, such as high blood pressure and hardening of the arteries.

• *Reproductive System Effects:* Decreased sperm count and sperm motility in male humans, and interference with ovulation in female monkeys. Considerable chromosomal abnormalities are found in mice exposed to THC. THC exposure causes some inhibition of male and female hormones that control sexual development, fertility and sexual functioning, which are reversible effects in sexually mature primates if drug use is stopped.

• *Immune System and Other Cellular Effects:* Possible interference with the body's immune response to various infections and diseases, possible mild immunosuppression. THC impairs the rate of tissue growth, leads to unnatural cell division, and produces cells with an abnormal number of chromosomes.

Other harmful physical effects include a reduction in REM sleep (causing users to sleep longer and not feel refreshed upon waking), and the exacerbation or cause of epileptic-type seizures.

EFFECTS ON PREGNANCY

Studies have associated use of marijuana during pregnancy with decreased fetal growth. Infants of these mothers have been five times more likely to have features similar to those in fetal alcohol syndrome (short and broad nose, flat face, narrower space between eyelids) than those born to non-users. The decreased fetal weight has been related to the amount of marijuana smoked, and has been greater than the weight decrease found in infants from alcohol-using mothers. Low birth weight is a major cause of infant death and increases the risk of illness. It is also associated with mental and physical handicaps, learning disorders, and behavior problems.

There is evidence that babies whose mothers smoke marijuana during pregnancy may have vision problems and shorter attention spans. Infants have increased tremor, startle, and cry responses. Also, the active chemical in marijuana, THC, readily crosses the placenta and is secreted in the breast milk, where it may further damage the breast-fed baby's development.

Infants of marijuana users may be damaged in two additional ways: an alteration in the chromosomes of the parents' reproductive cells could result in an abnormality of the offspring at the time of conception, where the genetic "change" could be passed on to the next generation; and a toxic effect of the drug on the fetus itself could cause organ or limb defects without changing the chromosomes.

Studies on animals confirm that marijuana contributes to slower growth in unborn babies, and show that high doses of the drug increase spontaneous abortions early in pregnancy and premature births or stillbirths later in pregnancy.

Smoking marijuana can affect the fertility of men and women and make it harder for some couples to conceive (this effect disappears once use is stopped).

DOSAGES

Users generally smoke from one to five joints per day, each containing 5-30 milligrams of THC. When a person smokes 100 or more milligrams of THC, memory and coordination are severely impaired, and the user may spontaneously fall asleep. (Joints contain from 0.5 to 1 gram of marijuana leaf, with a THC content of 1-2 percent. As previously mentioned, THC content in new strains of marijuana can be as high as 10 percent; in hashish 20 percent; and in hash oil, 85 percent.) The more THC consumed, the greater the psychological and physical effects. Marijuana from Hawaii, Thailand and certain areas of California is quite potent; Nepalese and Turkish hashish are thought by many to be the strongest "brands."

TOXIC EFFECTS AND OVERDOSE

While death caused by an overdose of marijuana is not a real risk, the drug can have many toxic effects, especially in susceptible people. Those at risk from even moderate doses include anxious, depressed or unrecognized psychotic individuals (who fall prey more easily to toxic psychosis and an exacerbation of psychological symptoms); heavy users of other drugs; pregnant women; some epileptics; diabetics; people with marginal fertility; and patients with chronic diseases of the heart, lungs, and liver. Adolescents may suffer from disruptions of hormone balance.

Chronic use can cause bronchial irritation and inflammation, a narrowing of breathing passages causing increased reactivity to irritants, reduced ability to clear the lungs, and possibly emphysema and lung cancer. People with heart problems may exacerbate or start angina pains through marijuana use. The immunosuppressive effect can leave a user open to a host of infections and ailments. Blood pressure elevation may cause strokes in susceptible people.

In the brain, cannabis can damage thinking, learning, and memory. High doses can create hallucinations and extreme anxiety. Long-term continued use may damage tissues of the brain.

Because THC remains in body tissues up to a month, effects on mental performance and the chance of toxic physical effects are increased and long-lasting. There is also the risk of a progressive build-up of toxicity in the regular user.

Cannabis is often consumed with other drugs, and it is this type of interaction that can cause fatal overdoses. Drug interactions can enhance or prolong behavioral, physical, and psychological effects of central nervous system depressant drugs such as alcohol or barbiturates. Cannabis has been shown to alter the effects of alcohol, barbiturates, benzodiazepines, nicotine, amphetamines, cocaine, phencyclidine (PCP), opiates, and other drugs.

TOLERANCE, ADDICTION, AND WITHDRAWAL

Marijuana dependency occurs when the user relies on the drug for support and cannot function confidently without it. Tolerance in heavy users builds rapidly. The chronic abuser may experience both psychological and physical withdrawal symptoms when he attempts to stop smoking, and this tends to perpetuate continued use. Withdrawal symptoms include: irritability, nausea, insomnia, loss of appetite, hyperactivity, increased REM sleep, and weight loss. These symptoms can last from 4-10 days. Physical addiction and increasing tolerance do not always appear in low-dose, infrequent users.

OPTIONS FOR TREATMENT

First, the physician must make sure no damage has been done by cannabis use and that there is not an underlying mental or physical disorder that the user has tried to medicate with marijuana smoking (e.g., anxiety, social phobias). A drug-free outpatient treatment program, consisting of family involvement, counseling, urine testing, and drug education is often successful. If, within a few months, the user is not completely drug-free, admission to a residential treatment center is advised. Several months are usually required to achieve a lifestyle free of drugs. When marijuana use is combined with abuse of other drugs, residential treatment is often the first step. (See Chapter Twenty-Four for more information about drug treatment programs.)

LONG-TERM PROGNOSIS

If use has not exceeded 2 years, most young people recover completely. Those with longer drug histories suffer difficulties with emotional and social maturation as well as long- and short-term memory problems, which often lead to relapses. Sixty percent of all people who try marijuana give it up after their initial exposure; 35 percent go on to use it once or twice a week; and 5 percent use it several times a week or every day.

Chronic use may cause permanent brain, lung, and heart damage. People can experience "flashbacks," not uncommon with hallucinogenic drugs, where marijuana experiences recur days or even weeks after taking the drug, although the user is now drug-free. These are rare in people who have not smoked any cannabis in over 6 months. Amotivational syndrome also disappears after months of abstinence. Long-term or irreversible effects on adult intellectual and social functioning are still uncertain.

CHAPTER EIGHTEEN

DEPRESSANTS:
Barbiturates, Hypnotics, and Benzodiazepines

Depressants, which also go by the name sedative-hypnotics, range from barbiturates to barbiturate-like substances to tranquilizers. Although their use has declined since the mid-1970s, they are still among the most widely prescribed drugs in this country. One out of nine Americans will take some kind of tranquilizer this year. Three-quarters will stop within a few months, but 15 percent will continue their use and may start abusing them.

One of the drugs we will discuss in this chapter, methaqualone, is no longer legally manufactured in this country—but its abuse still rose sharply at the end of the last decade.

Not only are depressants widely used and abused, they are also very dangerous. In addition to causing physical and psychological dependence, they carry a strong risk of overdose. People simply lose track of how many pills they have taken, or consume the pills with alcohol, increasing the potency of both substances. Because these drugs cause a quickly developing tolerance, one may need large doses to get "high," and only a little more to overdose.

Withdrawal from depressants (especially barbiturates and hypnotics) can be life-threatening. While withdrawal from narcotics can be a terrible ordeal, death is not common. People can die, however, when withdrawing from many types of depressants.

Depressants are drugs which, by depressing the central nervous system, will bring calm or sleep. They are generally prescribed to treat stress, anxiety, mental disorders, and sleeplessness, and some are valuable in certain cases of epilepsy. Legitimate medical use can evolve into a dependency problem if the patient takes more pills than the doctor prescribes. The addicted person may then seek additional "downers" through illegal means. People who abuse stimulants such as cocaine and amphetamines often take depressants to ease their frayed nerves and get to sleep. Narcotics users may resort to barbiturates when an opiate is not available, or to increase its effect.

Throughout history people have tried different substances to help them fall asleep. But there was no known synthetic substance for that purpose until the discovery of barbituric acid in 1899. This was the beginning of barbiturate research, although chloral hydrate, paraldehyde, and other bromide drugs were being used before the introduction of barbital in 1903. Barbital was the first drug that enabled doctors to employ the full range of depressant effects—sedation, relief from anxiety, sleep, and in some cases, even anesthesia. Since then, more than 2500 barbiturates have been developed, although only about 50 have made it onto the market.

Physicians soon recognized the ability of barbiturates to cause physical and psychological dependence, leading to the search for a safer depressant. Barbiturate-like sedatives were synthesized, along with tranquilizers. The first, meprobamate, appeared in the early 1950s. Unfortunately, these drugs were also found to be habit-forming.

The first benzodiazepine tranquilizer, chlordiazepoxide, was developed in the late 1950s. Diazepam, a similar drug in the benzodiazepine family, followed soon after. Since then these drugs have enjoyed enormous popularity. Although not as dangerous as other depressants, benzodiazepines can cause dependency when used regularly.

Barbiturate-like depressants were made as substitutes in the hope that they would be less likely to be abused than barbiturates and have fewer side effects. But the more effective replacements, such as glutethimide and ethchlorvynol, have proven no less dangerous and have their own harmful effects. Because it is more difficult to rid the system of these drugs than of barbiturates, their cumulative concentration in the system can make overdose more likely to be fatal.

Barbiturates have four types of effects—long-acting, intermediate, short and very short. In general, only the short-acting and intermediate-acting drugs have much appeal for the street user.

TYPES OF DEPRESSANTS

Depressants all have the same general effects with a few exceptions, although tranquilizers are much less potent and therefore less dangerous. The table on pages 158-159 lists all the types of drugs included in the depressant category, their approximate dose levels, and duration of action.

Long-acting barbiturates produce several hours of sleep. They can quickly build up in the body, resulting in a "hangover." Such drugs are prescribed for nervous insomnia, some forms of epilepsy and mental disturbance, and migraine attacks. The effects of these drugs start within an hour and last up to 10 hours. They are not commonly abused at the street level.

Ultrashort-acting barbiturates produce anesthesia within 1 minute after intravenous injection. This category includes drugs such as thiopental and hexobarbital. Their effects are not discussed in this chapter, because the rapid onset and brief duration of action makes them undesirable as drugs of abuse.

Short- and intermediate-acting barbiturates are the ones most sought after by abusers. After oral administration, they take effect within 15-40 minutes and effects last up to 6 hours. These drugs are prescribed for sedation or sleep.

Dependence and tolerance are most likely with the short-acting barbiturates, and withdrawal symptoms from these drugs are the most severe.

SEDATIVE-HYPNOTICS (DEPRESSANTS) OF ABUSE

Generic Name	Trade or Brand Name	Duration of Action*	Average Daily Adult Dose**
Barbiturates:			
Amobarbital	*Amytal*	Intermediate	no more than 1gm
Butabarbital	*Butisol*	Intermediate	15-100mg
Butalbital	*Sandoptal (in Fiorinal)*	Short-intermediate	50mg
Pentobarbital	*Nembutal*	Short	30-100mg
Phenobarbital	*Luminal*	Long	50-300mg
Secobarbital	*Seconal*	Short	100mg
Secobarbital and amobarbital	*Tuinal*	Short-intermediate	50-200mg
Talbutal	*Lotusate*	Short	120mg
Barbiturate-Like Agents:			
Ethchlorvynol	*Placidyl*	Short	500-750mg
Ethinamate	*Valmid*	Short	500mg
Glutethimide	*Doriden*	Intermediate	500mg
Methaqualone	*Quaalude*	Short	150-300mg
Methyprylon	*Noludar*	Short	200-400mg
Tranquilizers (Benzodiazepines):			
Alprazolam	*Xanax*	Intermediate	.75 to 4mg
Chlordiazepoxide	*Librium*	Long	5-100mg

Clorazepate dipotassium	*Tranxene*	Long	7.5 to 60mg
Diazepam	*Valium*	Long	4-40mg
Flurazepam	*Dalmane*	Long	15-30mg
Halazepam	*Paxipam*	Long	20-160mg
Lorazepam	*Ativan*	Intermediate	1-10mg
Oxazepam	*Serax*	Intermediate	30-120mg
Prazepam	*Centrax*	Long	20-60mg
Temazepam	*Restoril*	Intermediate	15-30mg
Triazolam	*Halcion*	Ultra-Short	0.125-0.50mg

Other Depressants:

Chloral hydrate	*Noctec*	Short	500-1000mg
Meprobamate	*Miltown, Equanil*	Intermediate	800-1200mg

Notes:

* Short is less than 4 hours; intermediate is 4-6 hours; long is more than 6 hours.

** Doses for children and the elderly differ; certain sensitive people react adversely to doses which do not affect others. Only a doctor can determine what dose is safe for a specific individual.

Not all brand names have been listed, particularly with the benzodiazepines. For a complete list, and more information about these drugs, see Chapter Twelve.

All benzodiazepines can cause dependence when used in high doses for a long period of time.

Non-barbiturate hypnotics can cause most of the same dependency and abuse problems as barbiturates, although they were originally believed to be safer. *Glutethimide* (Doriden) was introduced in 1954. Its sedative effects begin about 30 minutes after oral administration and last for 4-8 hours. Because the effects of this drug are long-lasting, it is very difficult to reverse overdoses, which often result in death. Taking more than 2 grams daily for a month can produce physical dependence. Because glutethimide is stored in the body's fat tissue, episodic release occurs, which may lead to periods of intoxication even when the drug is no longer taken. Unlike other central nervous system depressants, dilated pupils may accompany glutethimide poisoning. Overdosing on this drug has been implicated in suicides.

Methaqualone (Quaalude, Sopor) is a synthetic sedative chemically unrelated to the barbiturates or other hypnotics. It has been widely abused, partly because of its reputation as an aphrodisiac (due to the disinhibiting effects of all depressants), and has caused many cases of serious poisoning. It is administered orally and rapidly absorbed from the gastrointestinal tract. Large doses can cause coma, which may be accompanied by convulsions, and continued use leads to tolerance and dependence. Methaqualone and its chemical cousin, mecloqualone, are no longer legally available in this country.

The drug produces a sense of well-being, disinhibition, a "pins and needles" or burning sensation, unsteadiness, and lack of coordination. Some abusers take up to 2 grams a day. Deaths have been reported after a single dose of 8 grams, but most fatalities occur because the drug has been consumed with alcohol.

Methyprylon (Noludar) in doses of 200-400 milligrams will produce sleep. Prolonged use can lead to physical dependence. Six grams can cause death, but tolerance levels to this drug vary greatly.

Ethchlorvynol (Placidyl) is short-acting and its effects are felt rapidly. Physical dependence can occur with 2-4 grams a day for several months. The lethal dose varies, but 10 grams is usually fatal.

Chloral hydrate is the oldest of the hypnotic (sleep-inducing) drugs, first synthesized in 1862 and supplanting the then-legal alcohol, opium, and cannabis preparations for inducing sedation and sleep. It has a penetrating, slightly acrid odor and a bitter taste. Its depressant effects, along with the resulting tolerance and addiction, are comparable to those of alcohol, and withdrawal symptoms resemble delirium tremens. Chloral hydrate is a liquid, marketed in the form of syrups and soft gelatin capsules. Poisoning has occurred in cases where the drug has been combined with alcohol. Because its effects start to diminish so quickly, it is not a useful antianxiety agent, nor is it a popular drug of abuse.

Meprobamate, first manufactured in 1950, introduced the era of "minor" tranquilizers. It is an antianxiety agent and skeletal muscle relaxant. Its onset and duration of action are like those of the intermediate-acting barbiturates. It differs from them in that it is a muscle relaxant, is relatively less toxic, and does not produce sleep when taken at therapeutic doses. The usual dose is 400 milligrams three or four times a day, but chronic administration of slightly higher doses can cause physical dependence and possible seizures during withdrawal. The lethal dose varies from 12 to 40 grams.

The **benzodiazepine** family of depressants relieves anxiety, tension, and muscle spasms, produces sedation and prevents convulsions. While the margin of safety associated with these drugs is considerable and they have many valid therapeutic uses (see Chapter Twelve), overdose can occur (particularly when they are consumed with alcohol or other depressants). Continuous use of high doses for several months can lead to psychological and/or physical dependence. Withdrawal symptoms may develop approximately 1 week to 10 days after continual high doses of these drugs are abruptly discontinued. The delay in withdrawal symptoms is due to the slow elimination of the drugs from the body.

METHOD OF ACTION

Depressants slow down neurochemical activity in the central nervous system, with results that vary from drug to drug. The progression of effects starts with relief from anxiety and progresses to the suppression of inhibitions and then sedation. Sleep results at high doses, and large doses of certain drugs can even produce general anesthesia.

Disinhibition (decreased or lack of inhibitions) results from the suppression of the self-control mechanisms in the cortex and the release of impulses from the lower (and older) parts of the brain. This action is also responsible for the drunken euphoria and mood swings seen in users.

In addition to depressing brain and nerve activity, depressants affect the muscles and heart tissue similarly. They reduce the rate of metabolism in a variety of tissues and in the physical systems that use energy.

In normal doses, the sedative-hypnotic compounds appear to be selective depressants of certain pathways within the brain that are involved with wakefulness. The depression of synaptic transmissions within these pathways appears to account for the various stages of behavioral depression caused by these drugs.

METHOD OF ABUSE

Many depressant abusers started taking these drugs orally to relieve symptoms of grief, distress, tension or anxiety. Younger users, who also may inject the drug or consume large doses at one time, are looking for the euphoria or depressant "high" (the stimulated state of disinhibition euphoria). Some people take methaqualone purely for its disinhibiting effects. People may be self-treating social phobias or severe anxiety by abusing these drugs, when a physician could prescribe safer, lower-dose alternatives.

Depressants are sometimes taken with stimulants or with alcohol. Less popular but no less dangerous is the mixing of depressants with opiates. In addition, some methadone maintenance patients take depressants, claiming the drugs boost the effects of their medication.

Despite the growing unwillingness of many physicians to prescribe tranquilizers, few abusers have encountered much trouble getting the pills they want. But barbiturates have become scarcer on the street, and what is sold illicitly in place of these drugs is often either methaqualone or over-the-counter antihistamines. On the other hand, the street drugs called Quaaludes are rarely genuine. They are either manufactured in basement laboratories (along with many impurities) or are actually high doses of antihistamines or benzodiazepines, sometimes with 15 or more times the normal strength of these tranquilizers.

BEHAVIORAL AND PSYCHOLOGICAL EFFECTS

Users experience disinhibition, mood swings, intoxication, release of aggressions and hostility, sedation, sleepiness (although because of the disruption in normal REM sleep patterns, insomnia may also result from chronic use), "hangovers" after use, excessive dreaming, nightmares, euphoria, initial talkativeness, drunken behavior, slurred speech, lack of coordination, impaired memory, confused thinking, disorientation, tremor, and erratic movements of the eyes. People who take depressants may also suffer from extreme irritability, agitation, inappropriate behavior, and paranoia, sometimes accompanied by rage reactions and destructive acts. (The latter more commonly occurs when the drugs are combined with alcohol.) Slovenly behavior is often seen in chronic abusers.

PHYSICAL EFFECTS

Depressants have a host of minor physical side effects, including impairment of muscle control, erratic eye movements, and loss of reflexes. Methaqualone has its own additional side effects; among them are fatigue, dizziness, menstrual irregularity, skin problems, and a severe loss of muscle control. Paresthesia (tingling and numbness in patches of the skin) can occur, indicating the possibility of nerve damage near the skin surface, which can persist for months or even years.

Cutting down on depressants can cause a rebound effect that includes insomnia, headaches, stomach cramps, tremors, nausea, and vomiting.

EFFECTS ON PREGNANCY

Regular use of tranquilizers or barbiturates during the last months of pregnancy can cause the infant to have withdrawal symptoms, such as high-pitched crying, irritability, trembling, and sleep disturbances. Barbiturates have been linked to birth defects and may change an infant's or child's pattern of normal behavior and growth. Meprobamate can cause birth defects, and so should not be used during pregnancy.

A mother's use of sedatives and tranquilizers can make delivery more difficult and leave the newborn slow and tired. The baby also may have more serious problems, such as breathing difficulties.

DOSAGES

See *TYPES OF DEPRESSANTS*, pages 157-161. For barbiturates of abuse, dependent people often habitually consume amounts of 1 gram or more daily.

TOXIC EFFECTS AND OVERDOSE

Adverse effects on behavior are not uncommon. Patients who have underlying depressive illnesses may become worse—even suicidal— when prescribed these drugs for anxiety or insomnia.

In other cases, confusion after taking the therapeutic dose results in the ingestion of subsequent doses to the point of further confusion and finally overdose. Abusers can do terrible damage to themselves because of a lack of judgment, muscle control, and balance. Driving, swimming, operating any type of machinery (even common household items), getting in and out of the bathtub, and smoking in bed can result in accidents.

Barbiturates and their chemical cousins—but not the benzodiazepines—can alter liver function in abnormal and sometimes life-threatening ways. Any impairment of liver function affects every reaction in the body involving energy, including the detoxification of environmental pollutants and harmful chemicals (such as alcohol and other drugs) and the digestion of food. Depressant-induced changes in metabolism can lead to vitamin and hormone deficiencies and lowered calcium levels.

An acute overdose of a depressant can lower blood pressure and breathing rates to such a degree that failure to get immediate medical attention can result in death through respiratory failure or shock. Even quick medical aid may not help, since there is no antidote for overdose, and some drugs take a long time to leave the body. Death has also resulted from doses below lethal levels; when the "gagging" reflex is suppressed, people have choked on their own vomit.

Glutethimide (Doriden) has its own additional toxic effect on the central nervous system; it raises the heart rate instead of lowering it, increases body temperature, and causes convulsions. Methaqualone (Quaalude) can also cause lethal convulsions.

Moderate depressant poisoning closely resembles alcoholic intoxication. The symptoms of severe depressant poisoning are coma, cold clammy skin, weak and rapid pulse, and slow to rapid but shallow respiration.

TOLERANCE, ADDICTION, AND WITHDRAWAL

Tolerance to these drugs develops very quickly, which is why they are usually prescribed for short periods only when the doctor decides their use is necessary and no other drugs can do the job as well. For a short-acting barbiturate such as pentobarbital (Nembutal), tolerance to the hypnotic effects begins to develop within a few days, even at therapeutic doses. After 2 weeks, the effects are reduced by 50 percent. Cross-tolerance makes the use of other drugs from the same category ineffective, and using two drugs at the same time can result in accidental overdose. With chronic use, the liver enzymes that degrade the drug become more active; and the central nervous system cells adjust themselves to the presence of the drug.

Dependencies, both physical and psychological, can be created by all depressant drugs that are likely to be abused. Withdrawal is severe and more life-threatening than withdrawal from any other drug, so it should never be attempted without close medical supervision.

The abrupt cessation or reduction of high-dose depressant use can cause a characteristic withdrawal syndrome that should be viewed as a medical emergency. Initially, the patient may appear to improve. Within 24 hours, however, minor withdrawal symptoms appear, including anxiety, agitation, loss of appetite, nausea, vomiting, increased heart rate, excessive sweating, tremors, and stomach cramps. These symptoms usually peak during the second or third day of abstinence from short-acting barbiturates or meprobamate; with long-acting barbiturates or benzodiazepines, they may not reach this level until the seventh or eighth day of abstinence. It is during the peak period that major withdrawal symptoms may appear. The patient can suffer from severe epileptic-type convulsions. More than half of those who have these will develop delirium, often identical to the "psychotic" state seen in alcohol withdrawal. High temperatures may accompany these symptoms. Death as a result of respiratory or cardiovascular collapse is not uncommon.

OPTIONS FOR TREATMENT

Hospital detoxification is usually the rule for dependent depressant users. They are withdrawn by taking progressively lower doses of either the depressant of choice or a long-acting barbiturate, usually phenobarbital. When the drug the person has been using is employed—and this is normally the case with benzodiazepine dependency—he is started with a dose large enough to produce mild intoxication. The dosage can then be reduced by about 10 percent a day to avoid withdrawal symptoms. At this rate of reduction, however, sleep disturbances may appear, so some physicians prefer to reduce the amount more slowly.

Upon admission to the hospital, the pentobarbital or diazepam tolerance test is often used to ascertain the level of dependence. (This procedure takes advantage of the fact that cross-tolerance exists between the various central nervous system depressants.) Patients showing signs of depressant withdrawal are given 200 milligrams of pentobarbital orally. One hour later, the doctor examines the patient for signs of depressant intoxication such as sedation, lack of coordination, and slurred speech. If the patient is mildly intoxicated by this dose, he has probably been taking less than the equivalent of 800 milligrams of pentobarbital per day.

When phenobarbital (or diazepam) is substituted for the chosen depressant, it may take several days to find the right stabilizing dose, which is the starting point for detoxification. After that, doses may be reduced by 30 milligrams or more per day, and the patient is watched carefully for signs of either intoxication or withdrawal. The detoxification process may take 2-3 weeks or longer.

When a patient has a mixed opiate-sedative dependency, he is maintained on a sufficiently high dose of methadone to prevent opiate withdrawal while gradually tapering off the use of depressants.

Once the detoxification process is over, long-term treatment to avoid further drug abuse is the next step. If the drug involvement has been moderate, or if the drug of choice is a benzodiazepine or meprobamate tranquilizer, and there is little or no physical tolerance, no treatment at all or a mild outpatient program may be recommended. It is usually best to discuss the problem with a therapist to get a professional opinion.

If depressant use has been serious, the person may be self-medicating some physical or emotional disorder. This can be determined once the detoxification process has ended. If the person is suffering from organic depression, then he or she will be prescribed a more suitable psychoactive medication (such as an antidepressant).

A patient who has serious drug involvement and weaker personal resources is usually best served with residential treatment. This is especially true if he has an additional dependency on opiates or stimulants. If his personal resources are strong, then outpatient, drug-free treatment may be employed.

Former depressant abusers must find new ways to relax. Physical exercise, biofeedback techniques, yoga, meditation, and other forms of relaxation can help. Self-help groups such as Pills Anonymous can offer long-term support.

LONG-TERM PROGNOSIS

Few effects of depressants are permanent except for the nerve damage that may result from elevated levels of porphyrin, a chemical whose production is increased by the depressants' stimulation of certain liver enzymes. Long-term users may suffer from a number of medical problems and nutritional deficiencies, and damage caused by falls or accidents.

People who inject these drugs run the risk of contracting diseases such as hepatitis, heart-membrane inflammation, and AIDS.

Users with strong personal resources and/or swift and thorough medical treatment should recover from their addiction, particularly if the underlying problems causing the dependency are treated. Those with poor personal resources, or with concurrent addictions, show a lower rate of recovery.

CHAPTER NINETEEN

HALLUCINOGENS: LSD, Mescaline, and Others

Hallucinogens are drugs that distort the user's perceptions of the world. They are also known as psychedelics because they work directly on the chemicals and functions of the brain. Whereas delusions and hallucinations are hazards mostly to be avoided with the use of other drugs, people taking these psychoactive agents seek out their mind-altering properties. Some hallucinogens are natural and come from plants; others are synthetics, manufactured in underground laboratories.

The effects of hallucinogens are unpredictable and vary with the type of person using them, his state of mind at the time, his environment while using them, his expectations, and the type or amount of the drug used. In general, these drugs produce illusions of sight, sound, hearing, taste, or touch. They cause an inability to judge speed, direction, or distance. Sensory input of all types is exaggerated and/or distorted: colors may be "heard" and sounds "seen." Users may experience bad "trips" or good ones—either an onslaught of disturbing images with feelings of anxiety, disorientation, and alienation, or an insightful, almost "religious" experience of sensory appreciation and heightened self-awareness. Although high doses of all hallucinogens and even low doses of certain drugs are more likely to cause unpleasant experiences, again it is the mood and circumstances of the user that have the most influence on the nature of the hallucinogenic experience, or "trip."

The physical effects are generally not extreme. Pupils become dilated and the eyes are sensitive to light. Restlessness and insomnia may occur as the effects of the drug wear off. More serious physical symptoms include rapid heartbeat, rising blood pressure, and elevated body temperature.

Tolerance to hallucinogens is rapidly achieved, but this effect tends to limit use rather than increase it. Users may form psychological dependencies on these drugs, but no physical dependence or withdrawal syndrome has been reported.

Natural hallucinogens were among the first psychoactive drugs. The mushroom *Amanita muscaria* was used to produce altered states of consciousness in India in 1600 B.C. Peyote cactus (mescaline) was used in the New World long before the Spanish arrived, and the same is true of psilocybin mushrooms.

The modern age of hallucinogens began in 1943, when the psychedelic effects of an experimental synthetic drug called d-Lysergic acid diethylamide, or LSD 25 were discovered. During the years that followed, LSD was studied closely, mostly to see if it had any use in the treatment of mental illness. Some psychiatrists tried it on their patients, and government research was done to discover if it had the capacity to brainwash users. But it first achieved wide notoriety in 1963, when Timothy Leary and Richard Alpert, two young Harvard psychologists, were fired for using the drug with their students.

The use of hallucinogenic drugs began to grow throughout the 1960s, but declined after 1972. However, a second wave of popularity began a few years later; between 1976 and 1979, the use of psychedelics rose and fell again. Most of the early users of LSD and the drugs that followed it—DOM, MDA, and DMT—took relatively high doses and searched for profound experiences and strong hallucinations. By the late 1960s, this counterculture generation began to switch to the more natural, "organic" versions, such as mescaline and psilocybin. The second wave of users were different. They were generally younger, took lower doses of the drugs, and wanted sensory stimulation without potent illusions. However, phencyclidine (PCP) became a favorite among this generation, despite its disturbing and dangerous effects—the possibility of prolonged psychosis and violent behavior (see Chapter Twenty).

Because the drugs classed as hallucinogens differ with regard to action and effects, it is hard to generalize about them. Rather, each group must be examined separately.

⤴ LSD (D-LYSERGIC ACID DIETHYLAMIDE)

The hallucinogenic properties of LSD were first noted when Swiss chemist Albert Hofmann, accidentally absorbed a small amount through the skin of his fingers. The best known and most popular of modern hallucinogens, LSD is a synthetic agent derived from ergot (a fungus that grows on rye and certain members of the sunflower family). Ergot itself will produce hallucinations, and there are incidents of "ergotism" noted in history.

LSD is one of the most powerful of all hallucinogens, and its effects can be felt at doses as low as 10 micrograms, or one millionth of a gram.

METHOD OF ACTION

At doses of 50 micrograms or over, the effects of LSD peak in 2-3 hours, and can last for 8-12 hours. It is rapidly absorbed when taken orally, and just as quickly distributed throughout the body. Even a few micrograms in the brain produce psychedelic effects.

LSD resembles the neurotransmitter serotonin, and interferes with its normal action in the brain. The drug increases the sensitivity of the brain to all incoming information. LSD, psilocybin, and DMT (dimethyltryptamine) all resemble serotonin in chemical action.

METHOD OF ABUSE

LSD originally appeared as a colorless and tasteless liquid, carried in eyedropper bottles, sometimes wrapped in tin foil to prevent evaporation. However, the drug can be absorbed by many substances, and has been sold on pieces of blotting paper, sugar cubes, and small square flakes of gelatin. It has appeared as microdots (tiny tablets about the size of a pinhead), tablets, capsules, and powders of various textures and colors. The quantity of LSD in a black market tablet or microdot is usually between 150 and 200 micrograms.

Recently, individual doses of LSD have been put on sheets of absorbent paper which are divided into squares smaller than a postage stamp, printed with some type of motif or design, and which can be licked in order to ingest the drug. LSD can also be injected or inhaled, though these methods of abuse are rare.

BEHAVIORAL AND PSYCHOLOGICAL EFFECTS

The LSD experience can be very enjoyable or the complete opposite, and there is no way for the user to accurately determine which will be the case. About 1 hour after taking the drug, the user starts to experience profound mental changes. At very low doses (10 to 25 mcg) there is only a mild euphoria and loss of inhibitions. But with amounts over 50 micrograms, sensory perceptions are first heightened. Colors become brighter or change back and forth, tastes seem sharper, and sounds are louder, purer, and more complex. Patterns of color may appear, leaving trails around the environment. Time seems to stretch and perceptions of space and distance are distorted. Strange body sensations are common, with a feeling of floating or heaviness. Users become highly suggestible and can be emotionally manipulated. There may be dramatic mood swings, feelings of paranoia and anxiety, and a sense of detachment from the environment, from oneself, and from reality. Hallucinations are usually visual and can appear very real, although many users say they are aware of their illusory nature.

Forgotten events from the past, for better or worse, tend to resurface. Hidden joys or fears may emerge. The control over thought diminishes. The user may feel at one with the world, have profound spiritual feelings, or become terrified and disoriented.

PHYSICAL EFFECTS

The body reacts to LSD's effects on the central nervous system's receptors before the mind does, usually within the first hour after the drug is taken. Enlarged pupils, rapid heartbeat, shakiness, rising blood pressure, and elevated body temperature are common. Sweating alternates with chills, and breathing becomes rapid at first, then deeper and slower. Appetite may diminish, and some users suffer from nausea. Early effects mimic the "fight-or-flight" response to stimulation of the sympathetic nervous system, and agitation and insomnia may persist after psychological effects start to disappear.

EFFECTS ON PREGNANCY

Although more research is needed to pinpoint the precise effects of hallucinogens on unborn children, it is known that LSD crosses the placenta, so pregnant women are strongly advised against using this or any other type of hallucinogenic drug.

DOSAGES

The first wave of users preferred doses between 200 and 300 micrograms, although many took 500-1000 micrograms. At this level, adverse reactions were not uncommon, so second-wave users tended to take between 35 and 75 micrograms. Today, the average dose in most areas is around 100 micrograms.

TOXIC EFFECTS AND OVERDOSE

The most common toxic effect of LSD use is a bad trip. This can range from simple anxiety to full-blown panic attacks to toxic psychosis (with loss of identity, severe confusion, paranoia, delusions, and belief in hallucinations). Some psychotic reactions can last more than a day. Many doctors feel that psychosis that lasts more than 48 hours has been caused by the exacerbation of a pre-existing psychiatric problem, rather than directly by the drug. The same is true of severe and even suicidal depression; the drug may bring an emotional problem to light, but probably does not cause it.

Adverse behavioral effects are common. Users may feel they can fly or stop a car with their bare hands, resulting in severe accidents and deaths. Physically, none of the drug's toxic effects damage other organs, and even massive overdoses will not prove fatal (this is not true of the more chemically toxic hallucinogens such as MDA or DOM).

While experts once feared that LSD caused permanent genetic damage, they now believe the drug does not increase the incidence of genetic abnormalities or congenital malformations, even in people who have used it for extended periods of time.

TOLERANCE, ADDICTION, AND WITHDRAWAL

The tolerance that LSD produces tends to reduce rather than increase abuse. A rapidly rising tolerance (called tachyphylaxis) can become so great after three or four days of constant use that no effect can be achieved no matter how much of the drug (or of other similar hallucinogens such as psilocybin and mescaline) is taken. Sensitivity can be regained after a few days of abstinence. Compulsive LSD use is rare, although some early abusers did trip on a regular basis. There are no withdrawal symptoms when use is stopped, because the drug produces only a psychological dependence.

OPTIONS FOR TREATMENT

Most LSD users can find adequate treatment in outpatient clinics. However, if abuse has been heavy or prolonged, a psychiatric evaluation may be recommended. When psychotic reactions appear after LSD use, sufferers may first be "talked down" through reassurance and comfort. If unpleasant symptoms persist, a depressant for inducing sleep, or an antipsychotic or antianxiety drug may be prescribed. Prolonged psychosis is more difficult to treat, although drugs that raise levels of serotonin in the central nervous system are being tried, as LSD blocks serotonin receptors.

LONG-TERM PROGNOSIS

LSD appears to leave no permanent brain or body damage. Adult users who have not been taking other drugs should encounter little difficulty in remaining drug-free after a period of outpatient counseling. Younger abusers may need continued support to stay off drugs.

The most frequently encountered long-term effect of LSD use is the "flashback" where an ex-user experiences a repeat performance of hallucinogenic effects even though he is no longer taking the drug. This phenomenon strikes 5 percent of all users and 80 percent of all frequent users. Symptoms can range from mild distortion to episodes so severe treatment and sedation are required. Flashbacks rarely last for more than a few hours; they may only occur once or a few times over a period of months. No one is sure what causes them, but it is possible that certain actions or events—the use of other drugs (including alcohol), stress, anxiety—may trigger the nervous system to replay the hallucinogenic experiences. Flashbacks usually disappear within 1 year after cessation of drug use.

LSD-TYPE HALLUCINOGENS

There are several other compounds that closely mimic the actions and effects of LSD. Even though some have less pleasurable effects than LSD, drug abusers often take whatever drug they can obtain easily or whatever drug is given to them.

ALD-52 (Alpha-acetyl LSD) has almost the same effects and potency as LSD, but its actions start sooner. The trips tends to be a little "speedier" and commonly taken doses range from 45-90 micrograms.

LSA (D-Lysergic acid amide) is naturally derived from morning glory seeds. It has only 5-10 percent of the strength of LSD, but causes pronounced side effects (because of the alkaloids it contains) including nausea and diarrhea. It is also called ergine, and is taken in doses of 0.5 to 1 milligram.

Psilocybin and psilocin are found in about 90 different varieties of mushrooms native to Europe, North America and Central America. Psilocybin, which is metabolized by the body into psilocin, is less potent than psilocin itself, which has only 1 percent of LSD's strength. Large doses of dried mushrooms—from 5-10 grams—are needed to produce 4-6 hours of effects somewhat milder than those of LSD. (Six milligrams of psilocybin are considered enough to produce some psychedelic reactions.) After they are picked, "magic mushrooms" are either eaten raw, cooked, made into a drink, or dried for later consumption. Adverse physical effects include nausea, dizziness, vomiting, diarrhea, and stomach pains. Little research has been done concerning long-term effects. One danger of using these substances is that poisonous mushrooms may be mistakenly gathered and consumed.

DMT (Dimethyltryptamine), which is used in many South American snuffs, cannot be absorbed orally. It must be snorted or smoked (usually with marijuana), but it can also be injected. At 50 milligrams, it produces strong effects resembling LSD's that are more intense, but last no more than 45 minutes. Because of the short duration of action, this drug has been dubbed "the businessman's LSD," because a user can use it during a lunch break. DET and DPT are chemical cousins that may be substituted for this drug, though their effects can last up to 6 hours.

MESCALINE (PEYOTE)

Mescaline is extracted from the peyote and San Pedro cactus, found mainly in Mexico. This is dried and cut into slices known as mescal or peyote buttons. Mescaline was used by the Mexican Indians in their religious rites, and became known in Europe after the Spanish conquest. In those days, it was either chewed or boiled into a liquid for drinking.

METHOD OF ACTION

Mescaline belongs to the group of hallucinogens known as phenylethyl-amines and amphetamine derivatives, which includes such drugs as DOM (STP), DOB, MDA, MDMA, and TMA (also see Chapter Twenty-Two). These drugs are structurally similar to the neurotransmitters dopamine and norepinephrine (whose actions in the central nervous system they affect) and to the amphetamines (see Chapter Sixteen). When taken orally, significant concentrations reach the brain within 30-90 minutes. The effects of a single dose last for about 12 hours.

METHOD OF ABUSE

Mescaline "buttons" are either dissolved in the mouth and swallowed, or made into cakes, tablets, or powders, The powder dissolves in water and may be taken orally or injected. Usually more than one button is taken to achieve full psychedelic effectiveness.

BEHAVIORAL AND PSYCHOLOGICAL EFFECTS

Mescaline produces LSD-like effects including vivid hallucinations and impairment of color and space perception. Anxiety may also occur.

PHYSICAL EFFECTS

Common effects include dilation of the pupils, increased blood pressure and heart rate, elevated body temperature, and increased electrical activity in the brain similar to the effects of amphetamines. Nausea and vomiting often occur, but disappear after cessation of drug use.

EFFECTS ON PREGNANCY

See LSD.

DOSAGES

The most common dose is 200 milligrams, which is equivalent to three to five peyote buttons, but doses of up to 500 milligrams are taken.

TOXIC EFFECTS AND OVERDOSE
Mescaline is not considered highly toxic even in large doses, except for its possible effects on the digestive system. However, very high doses may rarely result in tremors leading to convulsive movements and physical collapse, sometimes followed by death.

TOLERANCE, ADDICTION, AND WITHDRAWAL
See LSD.

OPTIONS FOR TREATMENT
See LSD.

LONG-TERM PROGNOSIS
See LSD.

MESCALINE-TYPE HALLUCINOGENS
Synthetic chemical cousins of mescaline, also known as the hallucinogenic amphetamines, tend to be more toxic than mescaline itself. These drugs are explored in greater detail in Chapter Twenty-Two.

DOM (Dimethoxymethylamphetamine), also known on the street as "STP," produces LSD-like effects at doses between 2-5 milligrams that can last as long as 24 hours. Bad trips are not uncommon on this drug, overdose can be fatal, and there is the real danger of a DOM-induced psychosis that can last for years. Flashbacks occur frequently. Chlorpromazine may aggravate the unpleasant psychological symptoms. DOM is most commonly taken in capsule form. **DOB** is derived from DOM and is easy to produce. Although only one-tenth as strong as LSD, it is often sold as that drug, exposing users to the DOM-type dangers. The effective dose of DOB is around 2 milligrams.

MDA and MDMA, also known as "XTC," "The Love Drug," and "Ecstasy," produces effects different from LSD at doses between 50 and 150 milligrams. Users experience a serene euphoria, encouraging honesty, intimacy, and feelings of affection. At higher doses (between 150 and 200 milligrams) the effects are more like those of LSD; sweating, tension, and hallucinations may appear. Bad trips are rare at normal doses, but toxic levels (above 200 milligrams) can cause fatalities. Effects last from 8-12 hours. A new derivative of these drugs is **MDE** ("Eve"), which has similar effects.

TMA in low doses (from 50 to 100 milligrams) has the same effects as mescaline. At doses of above 250 milligrams, it becomes more like an amphetamine, and can cause hostile and violent behavior.

Myristicin and elemicin are found in the common kitchen spices nutmeg and mace. 1-2 teaspoons can be used to brew a tea, which after a 2-5 hour delay, induces euphoria and changes in sensory perception, including visual hallucinations, psychotic reactions, and feelings of dissociation. Unpleasant physical side effects include vomiting, nausea, and tremors.

OLOLIUQUI (MORNING GLORY)

Ololiuqui is a hallucinogenic drug obtained from the black and brown seeds of the Morning Glory plant, which grows in Central America and South America. It contains five closely related compounds that have properties similar to LSD. In fact, the seeds contain lysergic acid (but not lysergic acid diethylamide). It is one-tenth as potent as LSD, and its effects are similar to all LSD-type psychedelics.

The seeds are ground into a powder, soaked in water, strained, and the liquid is then consumed. About 300-400 seeds produce 200 micrograms, enough for an average trip. Physical effects are intense and include nausea, vomiting, headaches, increased blood pressure, dilated pupils, and sleepiness. Distortion of perception, hallucinations, psychotic reactions, and confusion may all appear. Flashbacks occur, but they are rare.

Despite its unpleasant effects, this drug is used because it induces mild euphoria and hallucinogenic experiences—and also, if it is the only thing available, a drug abuser may decide to take it.

PHENCYCLIDINE (PCP)—See Chapter Twenty

KETAMINE—See Chapter Twenty

BUFOTENINE (AMANITA MUSCARIA)

Bufotenine, found in small amounts in the poison mushroom *Amanita muscaria* ("fly agaric"), is a drug classified as a deliriant, a more toxic member of the hallucinogenic category. Deliriants are drugs of opportunity rather than drugs of choice; they are taken because they are available. Therefore, dependence is unlikely. They are generally shunned because of their high risks and unpleasant side effects.

Within 15-20 minutes after taking the drug, users can become confused and have difficulty breathing. Visual distortions, vivid dreams, and delirium are not uncommon. Increased blood pressure and heart rate, blurred vision, and muscle spasms are greater than those produced by psilocybin and DMT and are often very bothersome. Bufotenine can cause impaired coordination, minor paralysis, muscular rigidity, and speech disturbances. As the effects wear off, users may twitch for several hours and feel muscle pains for several days. Overdose will cause extremely high temperatures and prolonged delirium leading to convulsions, deep coma, and death as the result of cardiac arrest.

SCOPOLAMINE, ATROPINE, AND RELATED ALKALOIDS

These drugs, of which the strongest is scopolamine, come from the plants of the nightshade family and are also categorized as deliriants. They are used medically to dry secretions of the nose and mouth, and scopolamine has mild sedative effects. Users can take in substantial amounts by smoking jimsonweed, or by brewing jimsonweed or mandrake tea. The effects of these drugs, which are often taken with alcohol, can be alarming. Hallucinations, often of a highly unpleasant nature (i.e., monsters) seem real, and users lose touch with reality. A severe form of toxic psychosis can result, accompanied by prolonged hallucinations and excited delirium. Victims often must be restrained.

Physical effects include severe thirst, hot and dry skin, increased heart rate, and dilated pupils. Users may have difficulty urinating (this can last for as long as 48 hours). Accidents and falls are not uncommon, and overdose can result in death from respiratory failure.

These drugs are not widely abused. However, despite their drawbacks, some people use them because they produce euphoria, hallucinogenic visions, and feelings of flying. Persons may also abuse them because they are the only drugs available at the time.

Phencyclidine (PCP) and Ketamine

"Angel Dust," the common street name for the drug known as phency-clidine (PCP), is totally inappropriate. Given its potential for devastating psychological effects, "Hell Dust" would probably be a better name. Many experts feel that PCP poses greater risks to the user than any other drug of abuse. Psychosis and violence are often part of the lives of those who take this stimulant/depressant/hallucinogenic/analgesic substance.

PCP is a highly toxic drug that does not lend itself to low-risk use. It became popular with young users at the end of the 1970s primarily because of its "dissociative effect," the way it allowed them to detach themselves from reality. One adolescent abuser said that it made the world "look like TV."

Phencyclidine was investigated in the 1950s for use as a human an-esthetic, but because of its side effects of confusion and delirium, its development was discontinued. It became commercially available for use in veterinary medicine (under the trade name Sernylan) in the 1960s. In 1978, however, the manufacturer stopped production. Now, all phen-cyclidine produced in the U.S. comes from clandestine laboratories.

PCP is sold under at least 50 names, which vary from "Angel Dust" to "Crystal" to "Killer Weed." It is also frequently misrepresented as mes-caline, LSD, or THC. In its pure form, it is a white crystalline powder that readily dissolves in water. However, most PCP contains contaminants resulting from its makeshift manufacture, causing the color to range from tan to brown and the consistency from a powder to a gummy mass. Although sold in tablets and capsules as well as in powder or liquid form, it is usually applied to a leafy material, such as parsley, mint, oregano, or marijuana, and smoked.

Along with PCP, there are other precursor (those from which the drug is made) or analog chemicals being sold illicitly that have the same or even more devastating effects. The latter (analogs) are chemicals that are similar in nature to PCP—the only difference is that a molecule or two has been changed in the structure (see Chapter 22). The similar chemicals, created in illicit labs, include: 1-phenylcyclohexylamine, 1-piperidinocyclohexanecarbonitrile (PCC), N-ethyl-1-phenylcyclohexyl-amine (PCE), 1-(1-phenylcyclohexyl)-pyrrolidine (PCP or PHP), and 1-(1-(2-thienylcyclohexyl)-piperdine (TPCP or TCP).

A close relative of PCP, **ketamine** is an injected anesthetic used medically for special circumstances. Feelings of dissociation occur within 15 seconds after injection, and the patient loses consciousness after 30 seconds. Unconsciousness lasts for only 10-15 minutes, but amnesia persists for an hour or two and patients recall nothing they experience after regaining consciousness. Vivid and unpleasant dreams, as well as hallucinations, occur as the drug wears off.

When a user consumes a lot less ketamine than is needed for anesthesia, the effects can resemble those of LSD or PCP. The user may lose contact with reality and feel that he is floating in space. Ketamine has become popular among adolescents in recent years, and is sold under names such as "Special K" or "The Green" because of its color. It comes in the form of a powder, and is either sniffed or smoked. It is preferred by many to PCP for its briefer action and milder effects.

PCP used to be more popular with young people than it is now. When it peaked in 1979, 13 percent of the nation's high school seniors had at least sampled the drug. It is unique among popular drugs in its power to produce psychoses that resemble schizophrenia. Even a single dose of the drug can cause a toxic psychosis, often preceded by paranoid delusions and aggressive behavior. Although victims are usually violent—some law enforcement officials believe that the most heinous of crimes can be committed by a susceptible person under the influence of PCP—others become catatonic, and symptoms generally mimic those of an acute schizophrenic episode. In the case of PCP, any amount of regular use should be considered *serious* involvement.

METHOD OF ACTION

PCP is well absorbed when taken orally, intranasally, or intravenously, although oral ingestion is the slowest route to the central nervous system.

It is stored in fat tissue and brain tissue, so although blood levels peak 1-4 hours after ingestion, PCP can be detected in the urine up to 1 week following high dose use. The drug causes profound changes, possibly permanent, in the chemical balance of the brain, although more research is needed to pinpoint the reasons for its devastating effects.

METHOD OF ABUSE

PCP can either be snorted, injected, taken in tablet or capsule form, or smoked with substances such as marijuana. Some stronger "strains" of marijuana are actually laced with PCP.

BEHAVIORAL AND PSYCHOLOGICAL EFFECTS

The drug is as variable in its effects as it is in its appearance. A moderate amount often causes a sense of detachment, distance, and estrangement from the surrounding environment. Numbness, slurred or blocked speech, and a loss of coordination may be accompanied by a sense of strength and invulnerability. A blank stare, rapid and involuntary eye movements, and exaggerated body movements can often be observed. Auditory hallucinations, distorted body image, and severe mood disorders can also occur, producing in some users acute anxiety and the feeling of impending disaster, and in others paranoia and violent hostility. (However, stories of superhuman strength in PCP users are exaggerated.) At doses of 5 milligrams or less, the depressant effects are most often felt, with an alcohol-like intoxication and mild analgesia. At 5-10 milligrams, users may fall into a trance-like state. Any dose above 5 milligrams can have unpredictable psychological effects, and in susceptible people, even less may be needed.

PHYSICAL EFFECTS

Users may suffer from nausea, vomiting, cramps, insomnia, elevated blood temperature (giving the skin a dry and hot feeling), hypertension, and rhythmic movements of the eyes (up and down and from side to side).

EFFECTS ON PREGNANCY

More research is needed to pinpoint the precise effects of this and other hallucinogens on unborn babies. Laboratory animals exposed to PCP before birth have been born with severe deformities. Doctors believe this drug also may be very harmful to the nursing baby because animal studies show that PCP is concentrated in mother's milk.

Studies have shown that babies born to mothers who used PCP during pregnancy showed more emotional instability than other infants and were less easily comforted.

DOSAGES

At doses from 1-5 milligrams, PCP often seems like very potent marijuana. Above 5 milligrams, the effects are much less predictable. At 20 milligrams and above, hypertension, muscle rigidity, seizure, depressed breathing, coma, and death can all occur.

TOXIC EFFECTS AND OVERDOSE

PCP's negative effects on behavior are extreme. Accidental deaths can result from auto accidents, falls, burns, drownings (the hot and dry feeling of the skin causes many users to swim or bathe), industrial or household accidents (some users feel immune to pain and take senseless risks), and self-inflicted injury. Suicide, murder, and criminal arrests have also been reported.

Acute intoxication is marked by increased blood pressure, increased heart rate, rapid eye movement, sweating, drooling, and lack of coordination. Users may become agitated and violent, and develop full-blown toxic psychosis, which mimics schizophrenia. They may harm themselves or others.

There is a narrow margin between doses that produce the desired "high" of PCP and toxic doses, and they vary from person to person. Acute intoxication puts the user on the borderline of overdose. Toxic effects, both physical and mental, are difficult to treat, for there is no specific antagonist for PCP. As with THC, the drug is stored in the body for some time.

Overdose victims can suffer from extreme elevation of blood pressure, prolonged coma, and convulsions. Death may result even when timely and competent medical attention is available.

TOLERANCE, ADDICTION, AND WITHDRAWAL

While many PCP users do increase the amount they take, there is no clear evidence of tolerance to the drug. Physical dependency has not been demonstrated, although laboratory experiments with animals appear to indicate that such addiction is possible. Psychological dependence is created, and a number of abusers experience withdrawal symptoms such as physical distress, lack of energy and depression when they discontinue PCP use.

OPTIONS FOR TREATMENT

Patients intoxicated with the drug come to treatment centers mainly because they have aroused the concern of people around them. These patients are often confused and disoriented and may display bizarre posturing or even catatonia. They may seem anxious, apprehensive, or euphoric. Slurred speech is common and they often appear to stare blankly into space. Drooling, high blood pressure, and constant eye movements have also been observed.

Patients are placed in quiet rooms in isolation, to reduce any external stimulation, and restraints are used when the subject is violent. PCP users do not respond well to the "talking down" process, so care must be taken. Diazepam (10-20 milligrams orally or 2.5 milligrams intravenously) may be used to decrease agitation and muscular stiffness or rigidity. Most patients improve within several hours of PCP ingestion. However, that is not always the case. Toxic psychosis generally lasts for 3-4 weeks but may persist for months. Depression is also a common sequel to the psychosis. Antipsychotic drugs may be used (but not chlorpromazine, which appears to exacerbate the effects of PCP).

Any regular use of PCP must be considered profound involvement, and residential treatment centers are often advised. If personal resources are very strong, a drug-free outpatient program may provide all the help that is needed. Individual psychotherapy may also benefit the long-term PCP user, and self-help groups, combined with family support, are recommended by many for complete recovery.

LONG-TERM PROGNOSIS

Long-term PCP use can lead to anxiety, social isolation, severe depression, and violent outbursts. Schizophrenia-like symptoms are characteristic of some patients, whereas others develop memory and speech impairment. Many PCP abusers use other psychoactive drugs such as alcohol, marijuana, and different hallucinogens. These people are the hardest to treat. In general, the outlook for PCP users without strong personal resources can be grim.

PCP-induced psychosis may persist for a long period of time, although many doctors feel that this indicates a predisposition to, or a family history of, mental illness. The possibility of permanent brain damage remains an area of concern. Heavy users do show long-lasting mental impairment, including memory gaps, some disorientation, and problems with sight or speech. However, these disabilities seem to disappear within 6 months to a year after drug use ends.

CHAPTER TWENTY-ONE

OPIOIDS:
Heroin, Morphine, Opium, and Other Narcotics

When most people hear the words dependence, withdrawal, and addiction, they tend to think of the group of drugs known as opioids. The term *opioid* is used here to designate the group of drugs—both natural and synthetic—that are to varying degrees opium-like or morphine-like in their properties.

The picture of the wasted "junkie," propped up against a wall with a needle in his arm, malnourished and out of touch with anything other than where he is going to get his next "fix," brings to mind drugs in this category such as heroin. Unfortunately, as we have seen, there are many drugs of abuse that can put the user in the same situation. However, few have more dramatic effects and a higher incidence of rapid addiction than opioids.

Heroin dependency is no longer considered the urgent problem it was between 1968 and 1972, when use of the drug spilled out of poorer, inner-city areas into suburban America and onto the battlefields of Vietnam. Today, there are no more or less heroin addicts—about 500,000—than there were a decade ago. These numbers dropped off sharply during the mid-1970s, but picked up again at the end of the decade, when new sources of opium in the Middle East flooded the market with more potent and less expensive heroin. In addition, the invention of synthetic opiate substitutes, such as analogs of fentanyl (see Chapter Twenty-Two on designer drugs) that were created in underground laboratories, provided another cheap source.

While the use of these drugs remains heavily concentrated in poorer socioeconomic communities, the number of middle-class users is still significant. The popularity of cocaine has also affected the status of heroin, which has lost its stigma as a dirty, gutter-type drug. Some abusers of stimulants such as cocaine take opioids at the same time—a procedure known as "speedballing."

Opioids are used in medicine to relieve intense pain (analgesic action). They are also prescribed to treat heavy coughing, and for stomach disorders such as diarrhea and dysentery. Secondary to this pain-killing function, the depressant effect of opioids on the central nervous system causes drowsiness and may produce sleep; in street terms, this effect is called "nodding." Even though these drugs are widely used therapeutically, it should be noted that those derived from the opium poppy (also known as *opiates*)—opium, morphine, and heroin—are so powerful that continuous use will almost certainly cause physical and psychological dependence, even under medical supervision.

The relief of suffering, whether of physical or psychological origin, may result in a short-lived state of euphoria. That is the effect sought by users of these drugs. The initial reaction to these drugs is often unpleasant. Opioids tend to constrict pupils and reduce vision, and cause drowsiness, apathy, decreased physical activity, and constipation. A larger dose may cause sleep, but there is an increasing chance of nausea, vomiting, and respiratory depression—the major toxic effect of opioids. Except in cases of acute intoxication, there is no loss of motor coordination or slurred speech as in the case of depressants.

Tolerance and addiction to these drugs can develop within a week of regular use, and withdrawal symptoms are quite severe, though usually not life-threatening. Drugs such as methadone (which is a synthetic opioid and can also be abused) are often used to help in treatment, although a large number of chronic users never manage to get off the drugs completely and lead a normal life.

TYPES OF OPIOIDS

Opium

Opium has been written about and used for over 6,000 years. It was described by writers such as Coleridge, and was openly available as the medicine laudanum until the 20th century. While it continues to be smoked and eaten in its countries of origin—Afghanistan, Pakistan, India, Cyprus, Iran, Burma, Laos, Thailand, China, Greece, Mexico, Poland, and Indonesia—its impact in this country is most serious in its refined forms, as morphine and heroin.

Opium is a natural product of the opium poppy *(Papaver somniferum)*. Below the petals of the poppy flower is a sac or seed pod, which produces a juice during a short time during the flowering period. This juice is extracted by cutting a series of vertical or horizontal slits in the skin of the sac soon after the petals have dropped. The thick white juice oozes from the cuts, quickly coagulates, and turns brown.

The opium gum is collected and rolled into balls. This is raw opium, which has a strong odor. It contains morphine and codeine, both effective pain-killers. The poppy heads themselves are sometimes boiled in water to produce a drink that is a very weak solution of morphine (often below 0.2 percent).

Opium raw from the poppy is smoked, eaten or made into a drink. Raw opium is prepared for smoking by mixing it with water, heating and filtering it to remove the impurities, then further heating it to obtain the required consistency. When fresh it is like black syrup, but eventually becomes firm like putty, then hard as a lump of coal.

Opium that is smoked is either laid on a piece of tinfoil and heated (called "chasing the dragon") or placed in a special pipe. Opium can also be injected, and the effects are felt more immediately. However, not all injected opium is illegally used. It sometimes is employed in hospitals for the relief of severe pain.

At least 25 alkaloids can be extracted from opium. These fall into two categories: the phenanthrene alkaloids, represented by morphine and codeine, which are used as analgesics and cough suppressants; and isoquinoline alkaloids, represented by papaverine (an intestinal relaxant) and noscapine (a cough suppressant), which have no effects on the central nervous system and so are not considered possible drugs of abuse. A small amount of opium is used to make antidiarrheal preparations such as paregoric. Abuse of pure opium is rare today, unlike it was in the early 1900s when opium dens—establishments used for the smoking and drinking of opium—flourished.

When a person uses opium, he first feels stimulated, with enhanced imagination and speech. As respiration slows down, the imagination clouds, and thinking processes become confused. This leads to a deep sleep, and sometimes coma. As tolerance builds, more and more of the drug is needed for the pleasurable sensations, but the sleep has an increasingly rapid onset.

Long-term users deteriorate both mentally and physically. Loss of appetite leads to malnutrition, and dehydration results from vomiting. Blood pressure drops, and users feel cold much of the time. Stomach pains, severe constipation, and bladder disorders are not uncommon, and sexual and social drives markedly diminish. Infrequent users may have pleasant fantasies, but most often just become drowsy.

Morphine

Morphine, the main constituent of opium, was the first alkaloid to be isolated from the plant. It was discovered in Germany in the early 19th century. Morphine is extracted by dispersing the raw opium in water, then treating it with lime and filtering it. Ammonium chloride is added to the solution, yielding a crude morphine base. This is separated and further purified with other chemicals. The resulting substance is an analgesic, three to five times stronger than opium. Although it can cause sleepiness, it is mainly used to treat persistent pain and shock.

It is administered medically by mouth and injection, in doses of 10-

30mg. Its effects last about four hours. In addition to relieving pain, it can elevate the patient's overall mood. However, it may cause nausea. Street abusers can take the drug orally in tablets, inject it, heat it and inhale the vapors, or even use rectal suppositories.

Morphine is odorless, tastes bitter, and darkens with age. Only a small part of the morphine obtained from opium is used medically; most of it is converted to codeine or hydromorphone.

The euphoria produced by morphine can create an overwhelming urge to continue its use. An increasing tolerance, leading to physical and psychological dependence, quickly results. Side effects include nausea, vomiting, constipation, confusion, and sweating. There may also be fainting, sedation, palpitations, restlessness, mood changes, dry mouth, and flushing. An overdose is likely to cause respiratory depression and low blood pressure, resulting in coma and possibly death.

If a person addicted to morphine is denied the drug, withdrawal symptoms begin within a few hours, peak after 36-72 hours, and then gradually fade. Withdrawal symptoms vary according to the person and the degree of dependence. For some it is like a mild case of the flu; for others it is serious and extremely painful.

The most common symptoms of morphine withdrawal include: yawning, sneezing, irritability, anxiety, weakness, sweating, insomnia, nausea, vomiting, muscle tremor, stomach cramps, restlessness, muscle pain and cramps, and increased heart rate, respiratory rate and blood pressure.

Codeine

Codeine is also an alkaloid found in opium. It appears either as odorless, colorless crystals, or as a white crystalline powder. It is also a pain-killer, but with much less potency and mild sedative effects. It is either swallowed as tablets or used in cough preparations. It can also be injected. On the street, it is now being used with the hypnotic drug glutethimide (Doriden)—see Chapter Eighteen—in a combination known as "doors and fours," which produces heroin-like effects. Tolerance to this combination builds so quickly that users often take handfuls of the pills to get the desired "high."

Codeine, taken in doses of 120mg, can be used for the relief of moderate pain. Its effects last three to four hours. Side effects include constipation, nausea, drowsiness, dizziness, and vomiting. High doses can cause restlessness, excitement, and euphoria. In children, codeine can cause convulsions. If addiction develops from the prolonged consumption of very high doses, withdrawal is much less severe than from morphine.

Heroin (diacetylmorphine)

The discovery of morphine prompted the search for a new drug with the same pain-killing properties, but without the side effect of dependency. When heroin was first synthesized from morphine in 1874 by the Germans, it was thought to be that drug. The Bayer Company in Germany first started commercial production of the new pain remedy in 1898. It received widespread acceptance at first, and the medical profession did not recognize its high potential for addiction. It was not until the Harrison Narcotic Act of 1914 that it was first controlled as a substance of abuse.

Heroin is made by treating morphine with a compound that adds an acetyl group (two extra carbon atoms attached to five hydrogen atoms). Further chemicals are placed into this mixture, and by filtering and precipitation, the drug—which is five to ten times more powerful than morphine and the strongest analgesic known—is produced.

Heroin is the overwhelming drug of choice of narcotic abusers, but it cannot be legally imported or manufactured in the U.S. The dose taken by addicts varies—from 3 milligrams to 100 milligrams or more—depending on the person, the level of tolerance, and the purity of the product. Pure heroin is a white powder with a bitter taste. Street heroin may vary in color from white to dark brown because of impurities left from the manufacturing process or the presence of additives such as food coloring, cocoa, or brown sugar.

A "bag"—slang for a single dose of heroin—may weigh about 100 milligrams, usually containing about 5 percent heroin. To increase the bulk of the package sold to the addict, dilutants such as sugar, starch, powdered milk, and quinine are mixed in. Effects usually last from 3-4 hours, at which time the compulsive user must find a way to get more of the drug or else suffer severe withdrawal symptoms similar to those of morphine.

Most heroin addicts inject the drug, either by "skin popping" (injecting just below the skin's surface), or by "mainlining" (injecting directly into the vein). Effects are felt immediately, as the drug is carried through the bloodstream straight to the brain. Heroin is more rarely taken orally.

After regular use, the veins in the arms collapse, and addicts may then inject into the hands, legs, feet, even the breasts and genitals.

Heroin users first experience a sleepy, pleasant euphoria, and total relief from all stress and anxiety. After increasing use, a tolerance develops that makes it impossible for the user to feel any pleasurable effects at all. He must take the drug simply to avoid the pains of withdrawal. Among the side effects of heroin are appetite suppression and body dehydration. Hygiene is neglected, and "needle diseases" are common. Death can result from pneumonia, septicemia, hepatitis, jaundice, gangrene, as well as from an overdose. The new risk of contracting AIDS from shared or contaminated needles is a particular danger. Overdosing on heroin is more common among new users; long-term users build up a tolerance. However, no user can be sure of the relative purity of what he is shooting into his veins; the drug may be much stronger than he thinks it is, and overdose is the result.

Hydromorphone

Most commonly sold as Dilaudid, hydromorphone is the second oldest semi-synthetic opioid. It is marketed in both tablet and injectable form. While it is shorter-acting and more sedating than morphine, its potency is from two to five times greater than morphine. Therefore, it is a favored drug of abuse, and addicts usually obtain it through fraudulent prescriptions or theft. The tablets, which are stronger than available liquid forms, may be dissolved and injected. The most common dose is 1-3mg, and effects last four to five hours. Hydromorphone is prescribed for postoperative pain and to relieve the suffering of terminal cancer patients.

It causes less nausea and vomiting than morphine. When injected intramuscularly, it produces less euphoria, but intravenous injection will produce a "rush" much like heroin's. It commands the highest price on the street ($25 to $40 a tablet) of any illicitly used pill.

Thebaine

A minor constituent of opium, thebaine is the principal alkaloid found in another species of poppy, *Papaver bracteatum*, which has been grown experimentally in the United States as well as in other parts of the world. Although chemically similar to codeine and morphine, it produces stimulant rather than depressant effects. Thebaine is not used medically in this country, but is converted into a variety of therapeutically important compounds, including codeine, hydrocodone, oxycodone (see following), oxymorphine, nalbuphine, naloxone (see Narcotic Antagonists, page 189), and the Bentley compounds (mainly used on wild animals).

Oxycodone

This drug is similar to codeine, but is more potent with a higher risk of dependence. It is effective orally and marketed in combination with aspirin as Percodan for the relief of pain. The usual dose is 10-15mg and the duration of action is about four hours. Addicts take Percodan orally or dissolve the tablets in water, filter out the insoluble material, and inject the active drug.

Meperidine

Meperidine was the first totally synthetic opioid developed, which means that it was produced entirely within the laboratory; it was not derived directly or indirectly from opioids of natural origin. It is not chemically similar to morphine but produces the same type of analgesic effects. It is probably the most widely used drug for the relief of moderate

to severe pain. Available in its pure form as well as in products containing other medicinal ingredients, it is given orally or by injection, the
latter method being the one of choice for abusers. Tolerance and dependence result with chronic use, and large doses can result in convulsions
and death. It is better known under its trade name, Demerol.

Meperidine is given in doses of 60-100mg, but addicts have been
known to take up to 4 grams of the drug daily. The analgesic effect is
accompanied by mild euphoria, and duration of action is two to four
hours.

Side effects include nausea, vomiting, palpitations, dizziness,
headache, weakness, and constipation. An overdose can cause tremors,
involuntary muscle movements, dilated pupils and convulsions, sometimes followed by respiratory depression and coma. Withdrawal symptoms are similar to those caused by morphine dependence, although
they begin more quickly.

Recently, analogs (chemical cousins) of meperidine have appeared on
the street, and one tainted batch resulted in cases of Parkinson's disease
in the addicts who injected it (see Chapter Twenty-Two).

Fentanyl

A very powerful drug used mainly as an anesthetic for surgery, known
under the brand names Sublimaze and Innovar, fentanyl in analog form
has appeared on the street as "China White," and has been responsible
for a significant number of deaths from overdose. The medical dose of
this short-acting (30-90 minutes) synthetic narcotic is .01-.05mg.

Propoxyphene

Better known as Darvon, this synthetic opioid produces less analgesia
than codeine, but more than plain aspirin. With large doses, opiate-like
effects can be seen. The drug can be abused orally or by injecting the
powder, the latter method more commonly leading to dependency problems. The usual medical dose is from 60-120mg, and effects last about
five hours.

Methadone and LAAM

German scientists made methadone during World War II because of a
shortage of morphine. Although chemically dissimilar to morphine or
heroin, this synthetic drug produces many of the same effects. It was
introduced into the U.S. in 1947 as an analgesic and distributed under
such names as Amidone, Dolophine, and Methadone, but it became
most widely used in the 1960s for the treatment of narcotic addicts, a
function it still performs today.

The effects of methadone differ from morphine-based drugs in that it
has a longer duration of action (up to 24 hours), thereby allowing once-a-
day administration in heroin detoxification and maintenance programs.

Methadone is almost as effective when administered orally as it is by injection. But tolerance and dependence do develop, and withdrawal symptoms, although they come on slowly and are less severe, are more prolonged. Sadly, although methadone is used to control narcotic addiction, it is also abused and sold on the street, and has become a major cause of overdose deaths. Methadone maintenance programs to treat addiction are generally considered the last resort after other forms of treatment have failed; patients may have to remain in these programs for months or even years.

Methadone treatment is intended to be a temporary "bridge" to a drug-free existence, but some users find it hard to withdraw from the drug, even after several years. However, it is felt that a methadone dependency is preferable to heroin. This is partly because the withdrawal symptoms are less severe than those for heroin—hardly more than the discomfort suffered from a moderate flu.

Methadone users say the drug produces a "glow" milder than heroin's "rush." Among the drug's side effects are lightheadedness, dizziness, nausea, vomiting, dry mouth, and sweating. More severe symptoms include respiratory depression and low blood pressure. Circulatory failure and coma may follow, and deaths are caused by respiratory failure.

Closely related to methadone is the synthetic compound levo-alpha-acetylmethadol (LAAM), which has an even longer duration of action (from 48-72 hours), permitting a further reduction in clinic visits and the elimination of take-home medication. Its potential in the treatment of narcotic addicts is under investigation.

Narcotic Antagonists and Pentazocine

Scientific efforts to find an effective pain-killer that did not lead to dependence led to the development of compounds known as narcotic antagonists. These drugs block or reverse the effects of the opioids and have been tried (rather unsuccessfully) in the treatment of addicts.

Naloxone (Narcan) was introduced as a specific antidote for narcotic poisoning in 1971. Nalorphine (Nalline) was introduced into clinical medicine in 1951 and dubbed a narcotic agonist-antagonist. In a drug-free individual, it produces morphine-like effects; in a person under the influence of narcotics, it counteracts these effects. Narcan will increase breathing rate and depth, increase blood pressure, and dilate pupils. The problem with its use is that it may precipitate withdrawal symptoms within minutes.

A new narcotic antagonist, naltrexone (Trexan) became clinically available in early 1985.

Another agonist-antagonist is pentazocine (Talwin). Introduced as an analgesic in 1967, it was recognized as a possible drug of abuse. On the street, it was combined with the antihistamine tripelennamine as a substitute for heroin. Talwin, meant for oral use, could be dissolved in water with the blue antihistamine tablets—in a mixture called "T and Blues" or "T and B"—to produce an injectable solution. To prevent this misuse, in 1983, Talwin's manufacturers added naloxone to the pentazocine tablets. The new product, Talwin Nx, contains enough of the antagonist to counteract the morphine-like effects of pentazocine if the tablets are dissolved and injected. However, the drugs are still effective analgesics when used properly. The normal range of dosage is 30-50 milligrams, and the duration of effects is 3-4 hours.

METHOD OF ACTION

Opioids are readily absorbed from the gastrointestinal tract, nasal mucosa, and lungs, but intravenous use elevates blood levels and produces intoxication more rapidly. When taken intravenously, opioids are converted to morphine in the liver almost immediately. Peak blood morphine levels are reached in about 30 minutes. The morphine then rapidly leaves the blood and enters the body tissues where it concentrates. Only small amounts (about 20 percent) cross into the brain, but blood plasma levels correlate with the level of intoxication. All of the drug is excreted from the body within a 24-hour period (with the exception of the long-lasting synthetic drugs such as LAAM).

The opioids act by binding to specific parts of the brain and digestive tract (called receptor sites), triggering physical reactions. In the brain, the reactions produce drowsiness, relief of pain, cough suppression, and slowed breathing. In the digestive tract, they slow the movement of food through the system. These reactions probably mediate the action of the body's natural opioid peptides, the enkephalins and B endorphin, responsible for functions such as pain relief and appetite regulation.

Some scientists studying opiate receptors in the brain believe that the production of endorphins, which are the body's own morphine-like chemicals, drop off when narcotics are coming in from outside the body. When the supply is cut off, as in the case of withdrawal, there is neither heroin nor the endorphins to reach their receptors and trigger "slow down" signals. Therefore, a number of centers in the brain start transmitting at an accelerated rate. The autonomic nervous system, which controls breathing and digestion, begins bombarding its centers with confused messages that bring on such withdrawal symptoms as nausea, cramps, diarrhea, and flu-like symptoms.

METHOD OF ABUSE

Opioids can be taken orally, injected, or snorted. They are absorbed poorly when taken by mouth, although this can prolong their effects (which works well for codeine, methadone, and meperidine). Heroin, the drug that most easily crosses the blood brain barrier, is mostly snorted or injected, either beneath the skin or directly into a vein. Some users inhale the fumes off a piece of heated tinfoil.

A small number of heroin users manage to take the drug only occasionally for fun, or to take the drug cautiously enough to continue experiencing the same effects from the same size doses. This practice is known as "joy popping" or "chipping." But the majority eventually succumb to compulsive use. When heroin is taken regularly, tolerance develops over time, and more and more is needed to experience any euphoria. However, one danger is that tolerance does not always develop evenly—a user may need a great deal of the drug to obtain his pleasure, but very little to suffer from respiratory depression.

Eventually, the compulsive opioid user cannot get "high" no matter how much he takes. But he must continue getting the drug to avoid the pain of withdrawal. His life revolves around his use of the drug. Health and hygiene deteriorate. The addict may have to turn to crime or prostitution to afford his or her supply—chronic users can spend from $50 to $200 a day on the drug.

BEHAVIORAL AND PSYCHOLOGICAL EFFECTS

In addition to relief from pain and anxiety, opioids produce drowsiness, mood changes, clouding of the mind, euphoria, and feelings of peace, strength, and energy. The desire to do anything—include bathe—disappears with chronic use of these drugs. Addicts may sit around in a perpetual stupor, rousing themselves only when it is time to get more drugs.

PHYSICAL EFFECTS

While opioids suppress coughing, they stimulate other involuntary responses such as nausea and vomiting. Their ability to reduce the movement of food through the intestines makes them effective in treating diarrhea, but chronic use can cause constipation. Respiratory depression is another physical side effect, and can become quite serious with high doses of these drugs. Dizziness is also possible. Male users may suffer from diminished sexual capacity—the result of the opioid's ability to suppress the production of male hormones (which eventually returns to normal levels a few months after use has ceased).

EFFECTS ON PREGNANCY

When used by pregnant women, these drugs increase the chance of babies being stillborn or dying shortly after birth. Heroin addicts can suffer from a host of complications in their pregnancy, labor, and delivery. The babies of these mothers usually are born underweight and have difficulty breathing.

Babies of opioid-addicted mothers sometimes have withdrawal symptoms such as restlessness, trembling, disturbed sleep, sweating, stuffy noses, vomiting, diarrhea, high-pitched crying, and even seizures. These symptoms can start within 72 hours after birth and may last for 1-8 weeks. The severity of the effects depends on the amount of the drug used and how often the mother took it while pregnant.

DOSAGES

People have very different reactions to opioids, depending on their own metabolism, the type of drug used, and the purity of that compound. For normal dose levels, see the section called *TYPES OF OPIOIDS*, which begins on page 183.

TOXIC EFFECTS AND OVERDOSE

Nausea, vomiting, dizziness, and constipation are all common adverse effects, but the major toxic reaction is acute intoxication or overdose. This is normally the result of taking a larger or purer dose than the user's tolerance. Overdose may also result when opioids are taken too soon after a previous dose.

A person with a mild overdose may be stuporous or asleep. Larger doses induce a coma with slow, shallow respiration. The skin becomes clammy cold, the body limp, and the jaw relaxed; there is danger that the tongue may fall back, blocking the air passageway. If the condition is severe, convulsions may occur, followed by respiratory arrest and death. Although victims have recovered from respiratory depression only to die of such complications as pneumonia or shock, depression of breathing—often occurring with pulmonary edema (flooding of the lungs)—is the main cause of deaths. Antidotes for opioid poisoning (narcotic antagonists) are available at hospitals.

Because addicts tend to become obsessed with the daily chore of obtaining and taking drugs, they often neglect themselves and may suffer from malnutrition, infections, and untreated diseases or injuries. Among the hazards of opioid addiction are toxic reactions to contaminants, such as quinine (which can cause death from pulmonary edema), sugars, and talcum powder. Non-sterile needles and injection techniques, resulting in abscesses, blood poisoning, hepatitis, and AIDS, present another hazard. Accidents are not uncommon, and addicts often encounter violence, brought on by their own activities or from others.

TOLERANCE, ADDICTION, AND WITHDRAWAL

As mentioned, tolerance and dependency can develop very quickly. Withdrawal from opioids, while not as life-threatening as from depressants, can range from mild discomfort to pure agony. With the deprivation of these drugs, the first withdrawal signs are usually experienced shortly before the time of the next scheduled dose. Complaints, pleas, and demands by the addict are common, increasing in intensity and peaking from 36-72 hours after the last dose, then gradually subsiding. Symptoms such as watery eyes, runny nose, yawning, and perspiration appear about 8-12 hours after the last dose. The addict may then fall into a restless sleep. As the abstinence syndrome progresses, restlessness, irritability, loss of appetite, insomnia, goose flesh, tremors, uncontrollable yawning and severe sneezing occur. These symptoms reach their peak in 48-72 hours. The patient is weak and depressed, suffering from nausea, vomiting, dehydration, stomach cramps, and diarrhea. The heart rate and blood pressure are elevated, along with body temperature.

Chills alternate with flushing, and excessive sweating may be seen. Pains in the bones and muscles of the back and extremities occur, as do muscle spasms and kicking movements. The patient can become so depressed he becomes suicidal. Without treatment, these symptoms will run their course and most will disappear within 7-10 days. But for a few weeks following withdrawal, the ex-addict will think and talk about drugs and is very susceptible to relapse.

For some people, withdrawal is no worse than a bad flu, with the worst symptoms over in a few days. These people are usually addicted to lower doses or to poor quality narcotics (with low levels of purity). Some counselors believe that many withdrawal symptoms tend to live up to one's expectations. Withdrawal symptoms vary from narcotic to narcotic, but they are always unpleasant. Methadone, which is a longer-acting drug, has a milder, slower-starting but longer-lasting period of withdrawal than heroin. Withdrawal in most cases depends on how long a person has been taking opioids, how often he takes them, and how much he uses.

The abstinence syndrome can be avoided by reducing the dose of an opioid over a 1-3 week period, or longer. An addict can be detoxified by substituting oral methadone for the illegal opioid and gradually reducing the dose. However, because the addict's lifestyle is built around drug use, dependence is never completely resolved by withdrawal alone.

OPTIONS FOR TREATMENT

Opioid users, especially those who inject the drug, more often know they have a problem than abusers of other types of drugs. Unfortunately, many of them, and particularly the ones who come from poorer socioeconomic backgrounds, never seek help. Those who do should first go to a personal physician to see if drug abuse has done any physical damage or is covering up any chronic diseases. This doctor will probably be able to direct the drug user to a suitable program for detoxification and then longer-term treatment.

If medical detoxification is used, the patient will probably be given methadone. While some withdrawal pain may be present with this drug, the major problem will be emotional depression. In a hospital, the process can be over in 7 days; in outpatient programs, it can take longer.

In the past, the patient's daily maintenance dose of methadone (often as high as 70-100 milligrams) was reduced by 3-6 milligrams a day. However, withdrawal symptoms started to appear when the dose fell below 20 milligrams, and many patients complained of uncomfortable symptoms—ranging from insomnia to diarrhea—for months after the detoxification period ended. Today, many experts believe that methadone detoxification should last as long as 4-6 months.

There is great interest now in finding a non-opioid drug with which to safely withdraw opioid addicts. Clonidine (Catapres), an antihypertensive medication, has demonstrated some ability to relieve the symptoms of withdrawal and is being studied as a possible replacement for methadone. The most common adverse effect of clonidine is low blood pressure. There may also be a rebound hypertensive effect when the drug is withdrawn.

Antagonist treatment decreases the craving for opioids and their level of consumption goes down. Naloxone works for only 1-4 hours, but naltrexone works longer. An oral dose of 50 milligrams blocks the effects of 25 milligrams of heroin for 24 hours. The adverse effects of this drug include drowsiness, lightheadedness, nausea, and occasional feelings of dissociation from reality. On the whole, antagonist treatment is not well accepted by addicts, but it can be useful in combination with other types of programs.

Because physicians do not like to substitute a stronger drug with more potential for abuse for a weaker one, methadone is rarely used to detoxify abusers of pentazocine (Talwin) or propoxyphene (Darvon). Pentazocine users receive gradually diminished doses of the same drug, while propoxyphene abusers are usually detoxified with propoxyphene napsylate (Darvon-N).

One important thing to remember is that detoxification is only part of the treatment, not the whole program. It will help people get off drugs, but will not help them stay off. For that, a therapeutic community or a highly structured outpatient program is recommended (see Chapter Twenty-Four). Narcotics Anonymous is a self-help group that many former opioid addicts continue to rely on years after freeing themselves of drugs.

Some addicts are unable to abstain totally from opioid use. Chronic use may cause long-lasting or even permanent changes at the cellular level. This leads to a "hunger" that lasts for months or even years after withdrawal. The need to satisfy this hunger results in a relapse. For these people, methadone maintenance programs were developed. It was felt that medically supervised maintenance on methadone in doses high enough to satisfy the hunger was better than physical and psychological dependence on heroin or other illicitly obtained opioids.

Methadone maintenance entails the administration of 40-120 milligrams a day. Patients come to the clinic on a daily basis to get their "medication." Compulsory clinic attendance also makes the patient available for participation in group or individual counseling, which is a prerequisite in some clinics for receiving the methadone. People can eventually be withdrawn from methadone by a reduction in dosage of 5 milligrams per day.

Methadone maintenance has the highest success rate of any type of treatment for chronic opioid abusers. There are currently 75,000 patients being treated in this way, and 50-75 percent who begin this treatment remain in it for at least one year. However, it should be considered a last resort, to be used only when other forms of treatment have been tried and failed.

LONG-TERM PROGNOSIS

Opioids do not produce many direct long-term physical effects, apart from profound dependency. However, indirect effects include malnutrition and anemia, vulnerability to infection and diseases such as tuberculosis, "needle diseases" (AIDS, hepatitis, abscesses, endocarditis), and kidney failure and allergic toxic reactions caused by impurities and adulterants in street drugs.

The success rate of treatment for chronic opioid abusers is also not impressive. Those with strong personal resources can succeed, but strong personal resources are rarely found among high-dose, long-term abusers. In spite of urine screening, almost 20 percent of methadone patients abuse other types of drugs such as cocaine, amphetamines, and depressants. Alcoholism is an even greater problem: some studies have found that approximately 25 percent abuse this drug.

The successful treatment of chronic opioid abuse hinges on motivating the patient to seek an alternative lifestyle to one dominated by drugs. Remedial education, job training and placement, legal assistance, and individual, group, and family counseling should supplement any other type of treatment in order to keep the ex-addict drug-free for the rest of his or her life.

CHAPTER TWENTY-TWO
Designer Drugs

The increasing demand on the street for psychoactive drugs over the past two decades has led to a proliferation of illicit clandestine laboratories. They can be located anywhere—in basements, garages, warehouses, apartments or private homes. With limited chemical knowledge and relatively cheap materials, operators of underground laboratories can concoct large batches of illegal chemicals such as hallucinogens, amphetamines, and depressants.

These labs are hard to find. Many drug enforcement agencies have been set up to stop the flow of drugs into this country, but they have limited resources to deal with labs within our borders. Clandestine drug factories have produced almost two dozen kinds of controlled substances, some with dangerous chemical adulterants and others so potent that one dose can cause immediate death.

Designer drugs is the term given to drugs from illicit laboratories that are synthetic look-alike and act-alike spinoffs (called analogs) of high demand drugs such as heroin. They are chemically designed—altered by one or two molecules in the original drug formula—to be more potent, to be cheaper, or to sidestep restrictions on the original drug's use and sale. There is an almost endless parade of subtly different preparations that can be obtained from a single chemical formula simply by switching a few molecular links in a drug family chain.

Designer drugs can be manufactured in illicit labs by anyone with a small investment in glassware and an even smaller acquaintance with chemistry. Huge profits can be made by people with an extra $500 and a college chemistry course or two under their belts.

Most lab operators make the illicit drugs from formulas found in underground drug cookbooks or recipes handed down by friends. The enterprising few who make designer varieties of amphetamines, PCP, hallucinogens, and heroin substitutes usually take these formulas from scientific journals. Often, drug companies make several analogs of a chemical agent to test potency and feasibility of manufacture. They may never use these analogs, but the formulas for them are on record.

No one knows how many possible weird, new chemical concoctions are out there or will turn up in the future—or how many users will be seriously harmed or killed by taking them. It has been theorized that one underground chemist with the right supplies could make enough heroin to supply the entire world's demands without ever harvesting a single opium poppy. Designer drugs represent a new—and very dangerous—problem in the world of illicit drug use.

FENTANYL ANALOGS

In 1980, the first hint of designer disaster appeared on the West Coast when a new type of heroin turned up on the streets. It took 10 months and some 30 overdose deaths later for chemists of the DEA (Drug Enforcement Administration) to track it down. Sold as "China White," a highly potent form of Southeast Asian heroin, it looked just like the real thing but didn't test as heroin in urine and blood samples taken from the victims. DEA chemists kept working and finally discovered that the drug wasn't an opiate-based narcotic, but alpha-methylfentanyl (AMF), a little-known and easily made relative of the surgical anesthetic fentanyl. (Fentanyl is a synthetic narcotic sold as Sublimaze and Innovar, which is used in major surgery.) This event marked the first time anyone had made or sold legal heroin substitutes on a large scale.

Later, a new analog was discovered: 3-Methylfentanyl. Both drugs differed from the parent compound by the attachment of a single methyl group (see Figure 6). This methyl group attached to a particular site on the molecule and changed the structure just enough to make the drug as legal as hamburgers.

In May 1981, the DEA authorities came across para-fluorofentanyl. This stunned them, because unlike alpha-methyl fentanyl and 3-Methylfentanyl, it had never been written up in the open literature. The manufacture of a unique compound meant that a talented chemist was at work in this field, and such a situation could easily spell disaster. If clandestine labs started making designer heroins in earnest and dealers switched to these drugs, the country could be overrun with cheap, legal, heroin substitutes, leading to an epidemic of addiction and overdose. There may indeed be thousands of analogs of fentanyl which can be made by a chemist with more advanced knowledge.

Drugs from the fentanyl series work well as heroin substitutes because they work just like heroin: they block pain and cause euphoria by binding to opiate receptors in the brain. However, the potency is very different, and that is what caused the overdose deaths. Fentanyl is 100 times as strong as morphine. Some of the illegally produced analogs are so potent that 1 gram is enough to make 50,000 doses (which is about 250 times stronger than heroin). Some doctors have estimated that 300 mcg of either fentanyl compound would be enough to shut down respiration and kill a novice user who had not built up any tolerance.

FIGURE 6
Synthetic (Designer) Narcotics—Fentanyl Analogs

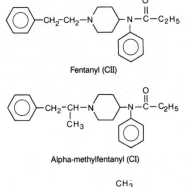

Fentanyl (CII)

Alpha-methylfentanyl (CI)

3-Methylfentanyl (CI)

The narcotic analogs of the surgical anesthetic fentanyl are so similar in structure to the parent drug that it is hard to tell the difference at first glance.

Underground chemists rarely test the potency of a drug in normal ways. Instead, they give "free samples" to users on the street and watch the effects. Sometimes they don't even do that.

In fact, potency is the key to profits with designer drugs. Some chemists at the DEA believe that these labs manufacture the analogs not so much because they are legal for a short time (until the government authorities discover them and makes new adjustments in the law), but because the increased strength can produce so much for so little. About $200 worth of starter chemicals (bought in illegal supply houses) can produce a two-year supply that retails for up to $2 million. But the high potency of the drugs make it difficult to dilute a dose (with standard cuts such as lactose) to a safe consistency.

Because fentanyl's respiratory-depressant effects are longer-lasting than its narcotic effects, when overdose does occur, it requires immediate medical attention. Sometimes even that cannot save a person's life. Since China White's debut in late 1979, it has killed almost 100 people and continues to kill at the rate of two per month.

The fentanyl drugs are at this point mainly a West Coast problem, but one which seems to be spreading. It is estimated that 20 percent of Californian addicts are hooked on designer heroin. Because the chemical does not show up in drug tests unless it is specifically suspected and tested for, there may be many unreported deaths, as well as chronic users who pass screening tests even though they regularly use the drugs.

The action, methods of abuse, effects, tolerance levels, addiction, withdrawal and treatment of synthetic narcotic abuse are approximately the same as for opiate-based narcotics (see Chapter Twenty-One). Synthetic drugs primarily act on the central nervous system and the gastrointestinal tract. In addition to producing analgesia (relief from pain), drowsiness and euphoria, these substances can also cause varying degrees of respiratory depression, constipation, muscular rigidity, and changes in the autonomic nervous system.

MEPERIDINE ANALOGS

As bad as street fentanyl is, an underground chemist in 1982 rushed his recipe for a heroin substitute, missed by a long shot, and made something even worse. Working backward from a government listing of synthetic painkillers, the chemist found a still legal psychoactive analog of meperidine (Demerol), a prescription drug used to relieve pain. Impatient with the slow "cooking time" needed to produce the analog, called 1-methyl-4-phenyl-4-propionoxypiperidine (MPPP), he added extra acid and turned up the heat to speed the processing (See Figure 7). These shortcuts backfired, and when heroin addicts injected this new batch of "China White" or "new heroin," they short-circuited their central nervous systems.

What slipped into the unfortunate batch of synthetic narcotics was an unwanted chemical by-product and contaminant called 1-methyl, 4-phenyl-1, 2,5,6-tetrahydropyridine (MPTP). It caused an incurable syndrome, characterized by permanent and progressive brain and nervous system damage and almost complete paralysis. It was similar to Parkinson's disease, which is a chronic, progressive, central nervous system disorder characterized by slowness and lack of purposeful movements, muscular rigidity, and tremor. People who used this drug were later called "frozen addicts," because many of them literally froze in place, some with the needles still stuck in their arms. Others gradually came down with the disease in a few days. The typical user suffered as much brain damage in two to three doses as if he had suffered from the progressive effects of Parkinson's disease for ten years. In many cases, the symptoms appeared 2-10 days after use, starting with arthritis-type problems, including stiffness, tremors, seizures, and difficulty in speaking.

FIGURE 7
Synthetic (Designer) Narcotics—Meperideine Analogs

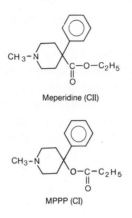

Meperidine (CII)

MPPP (CI)

Batches of contaminated MPPP (an analog of meriperidine) have caused permanent brain and nervous system damage in users.

This synthetic heroin was described as a sticky brown powder and it surfaced again in 1983. Reports of drug-induced Parkinson's disease have been reported as far away as British Columbia. The only way users can recognize the drug as this particularly harmful synthetic is by the burning sensation it leaves *after* injection.

Symptoms of Parkinson's disease appear whenever the brain's supply of dopamine, a crucial neurotransmitter, is interrupted. If the brain runs short on dopamine, neural signals that instruct the muscles to work get lost or blocked. No one knows what exactly causes the disease (although ironically, the tragedy with MPTP has helped researchers in the field understand more about Parkinson's disease), but it almost always strikes older adults—one person out of 100 between the ages of 60 and 65.

When people suffering from the disease are treated with L-dopa, the substance the brain converts to dopamine, the symptoms are somewhat alleviated. Frozen addicts who were given this drug did indeed "melt," but the problem with L-dopa therapy is that over time the drug becomes less effective in reversing the paralysis. As soon as these addicts were taken off the drug, they froze up again.

In the classical form of the disease, extensive cell death occurs in the substantia nigra, a crucial dopamine pathway of the brain. Doctors from the National Institutes of Mental Health found identical damage in the brains of drug abusers who used the faulty MPPP. When researchers searched for more information about MPPP in the Stanford University library, they found that all relevant articles had been razored out of the journals, probably taken by an illegal drug manufacturer. They did find that MPTP was a powerful neurotoxin, which caused Parkinson's disease in monkeys who were injected with a few milligrams of the chemical. The meperidine analog MPPP, first identified by DEA labs in 1982, is about five to ten times more potent as an analgesic than meperidine and is similar to morphine.

The chronic use of meperidine has other toxic side effects, including tremors, muscle twitches, hallucinations, seizures, and nausea. The dangers associated with the use of all opiate-based and synthetic narcotics also hold for meperidine analog abuse.

Another meperidine analog, 1-(2-phenylethyl)-4-acetyloxypiperidine (PEPAP) was detected in 1985 from samples analyzed by the DEA laboratory system. The samples also contained a by-product that is chemically related to the neurotoxin MPTP. As with fentanyl, there may be many more analogs of meperidine waiting to be discovered by underground chemists.

HALLUCINOGENIC AMPHETAMINES

Several dozen analogs of amphetamine and methamphetamine are hallucinogenic and have appeared on the street over the past two decades. The actions of the derivatives of amphetamine (MDA, DMA, PMA, TMA, MMDA), methamphetamine (MDMA) and phenethylamine (mescaline, BDMPEA) are somewhat similar: they all tend to produce mescaline-like behavior (see Chapter 19). At lower doses, there is increased motor activity, increased sensory perception, analgesia, and varying levels of intoxication. Users may experience euphoria or fright, sensory distortions or hallucinations, nausea, vomiting, jaw clenching, flushing, increased blood pressure, enlarged pupils, impaired balance and a loss of coordination. With increasing amounts, muscle rigidity, tremors, convulsions, and death can all occur.

The amphetamine analogs currently of the most concern are 3,4-methylenedioxyamphetamine (MDA) and 3,4-methylenedioxymethamphetamine (MDMA). MDA was one of the most sought-after drugs of the 1960s, first appearing in San Francisco in 1967. It gained a reputation for producing a sensual, easily managed euphoria, and was nicknamed the "love drug." However, studies found that a single high dose administered to a rat (normally above 150 milligrams in a human) could cause permanent brain damage. In recent years, this drug and its chemical cousin, MDMA, have emerged as the "yuppie psychedelics."

MDMA, more popularly known as XTC, Ecstasy, or Adam, has received considerable attention from the media. It is reported to be very popular on college campuses for its euphoric properties, and in the early

1980s, some doctors prescribed it for patients as an adjunct to psychotherapy, although studies have not been done on its safety and effectiveness. Doctors who have employed the drug in treatment report that it helps patients express their feelings, communicate better, and resolve painful emotional problems.

In July, 1985, MDMA was placed in Schedule I (the strongest category) of the Controlled Substances Act, carrying the most severe penalties for its illegal use and trafficking. This is because MDMA, in addition to producing euphoria, can also cause confusion, depression, anxiety, and paranoia. Physical symptoms include muscle tension, nausea, blurred vision, liver problems, faintness, chills, or sweating. It also increases the heart rate and blood pressure.

"Ecstasy" costs about $10 per dose, and its effects last from 8-12 hours. The usual effective dose is from 100-150 milligrams taken orally, but some people have been known to abuse the drug in smaller doses from 10-15 times a day.

Both MDA and MDMA appear to affect dopamine and norepinephrine by releasing them from their nerve terminals and blocking re-uptake. They also seem to affect serotonin in many ways. MDMA, has been shown to destroy serotonin-producing neurons in animals. These neurons play a direct role in regulating aggression, mood, sexual activity, sleep, and sensitivity to pain. In animal studies, the doses of MDA that can damage these serotonergic nerve cells are only two to three times more than minimum dosages needed to produce euphoric effects. What this means to human behavior is still under investigation.

On the street, MDA, MDMA—and a still newer spinoff, MDE ("Eve")—are usually sold as a white or gray-white powder that can be inhaled, injected, or swallowed. While the physical effects are similar to those produced by amphetamines (see Chapter Sixteen), users describe feelings of calm, heightened sensitivity, and increased insight. These drugs typically produce less dissociation and disorientation and fewer anxiety reactions than psychedelics.

Other hallucinogenic amphetamines are more harmful than MDA and MDMA. PMA and DOM (also called STP) can trigger panic and anxiety attacks, often lasting for hours or days. PMA is highly toxic, and a fatal dose is equal to a mild dose of mescaline. DOB is known to produce spasms in blood vessels that can completely shut off blood flow to the arms and legs.

These drugs differ from one another in their speed of onset, duration of action, potency, and capacity to modify mood, with or without producing hallucinations. They are usually taken orally and sometimes snorted, but rarely injected. Because all are produced in clandestine laboratories, they are seldom pure, and the dose (in a tablet, capsule, or on a square of impregnated paper) can vary considerably. In general, users experience disturbances in direction, time and distance, mood alterations (from euphoria to depression), and sometimes delusions and hallucinations. The depression and feelings of estrangement from one's surroundings can become so severe that suicide is possible. Impaired judgment can lead to accidents of all types. Users may also suffer from "flashbacks," where the psychedelic feelings recur even when the drug is no longer being used.

The use of hallucinogenic amphetamines can lead to tolerance and overdose, although the dependence appears to be mainly psychological.

OTHER ANALOGS

The new designer heroins and hallucinogenic amphetamines are only the most recent additions to the host of synthetic drugs produced in illicit labs. Other frequently found drug analogs include:

- *Phencyclidine analogs* (PCE, TCP, PHP, PCC). All more potent but with the same general effects as PCP (see Chapter Twenty).
- *Short-acting hallucinogens* (including the hallucinogen DMT and its analogs DET and DPT). Best known for their sudden, intense hallucinogenic affects.
- *Methaqualone analog* (mecloqualone). Effects similar to the parent compound.

Analogs of drugs are certainly not restricted to illicit manufacture and use. Witness the large number of variations on a theme found within the benzodiazepine family (see Chapter Twelve) in which the "parent" drug is chlordiazepoxide (Librium). Although all drugs in a family are similar in chemical structure and action, they have slight differences in their chemical makeup, which is why one drug in a family might work better on one person than another.

Some illegal drugs such as cocaine are presently too difficult and expensive to make in a laboratory. Manufacturing morphine from scratch would cost more than the street price of regular morphine— hence, an analog of fentanyl is used instead.

Other drugs, such as marijuana, have increased in potency through modern methods of plant breeding and cultivation. Marijuana in the 1960s had an average concentration of 1-3 percent THC, whereas many batches today have a THC concentration of over 10 percent.

As technology and procedures advance during the coming years, researchers and law enforcement officials hope that new methods of synthesizing illegal drugs will not appear at the same time, flooding the market with cheap and easily obtained "copies," causing a major drug epidemic.

DANGERS OF CHEMICAL ALTERATION

Drugs can be made even more dangerous in illicit laboratories through the use of the following procedures:

- *Dilution*, which increases bulk and reduces purity, through the use of inert materials such as talc, flour, cornstarch, and sugars such as mannitol, lactose, dextrose, sucrose, and inositol. These can cause added physical side effects. Abrasive additives can aggravate the damage cocaine does to the nasal passages, and produce real risks for the intravenous user.
- *Adulteration*, which occurs when the drug is cut with active ingredients such as caffeine and ephedrine, or local anesthetics such as lidocaine and benzocaine. These substances can add to the physical and psychological effects of the original drug. Marijuana may be spiked with PCP and passed off as high-quality pot. In cases like this, the user will experience symptoms he does not expect or want.
- *Contamination*, which is best illustrated by the case of the MPPP that yielded the neurotoxic by-product, MPTP. Residues of potassium cyanide have been found in samples of both PCP and illicitly manufactured methamphetamine.

Clearly, one of the newest dangers of purchasing drugs "on the street" is that the user doesn't know enough about the drug he is buying, how much of it he is taking, and what other poisonous chemicals he may be consuming when he takes it. He may not even be getting what he thought he purchased. Substitution, the practice of selling one drug but calling it another drug, is not uncommon in illicit markets. LSD is often sold as psilocybin or mescaline. When the user gets a more powerful drug than the one he bargained for, panic and unexpected psychological damage can ensue.

CHAPTER TWENTY-THREE

Inhalants, Solvents, and Other Volatile Substances

The increase in the abuse of volatile solvents and aerosols, as well as inhalants such as amyl and butyl nitrate, is a recent phenomenon that mainly affects young children and adolescents. It can quickly lead to severe psychological dependence. Boys in their young teens, particularly from areas where money for more expensive drugs is scarce, are the most vulnerable. Although this type of drug use is normally a passing fad of youth, volatile solvents and aerosols are the most physically threatening of all psychoactive drugs. They can leave the user with permanent brain, kidney and liver damage, and may lead to certain types of leukemia. Accidental death is also not uncommon.

The popular term "glue sniffing" is too limited, because inhalant abuse can involve many household substances, from paint thinners to antifreeze to hair sprays. It has been estimated that the average household has more than 30 substances that can be abused.

In ancient Greece, the Priestess at the Oracle of Delphi inhaled fumes (probably carbon dioxide) from crevices in the rocks, so that she would have "visions" of a prophetic nature. Laughing gas (nitrous oxide) was produced in the late 1800s and often abused as a recreational drug because of its euphoric effects. Chloroform and ether soon joined the list, and solvent abuse as we know it first appeared in the 1950s. Amyl and butyl nitrate became popular in the 1960s, largely for their reputation of enhancing sex. (Previously, amyl nitrate was used to relieve the symptoms of angina pectoris by lowering the resistence of blood vessels, so lessening the strain on the heart.) Gasoline was the first solvent abused on a wide scale, and model glue became popular soon afterward. Aerosols were misused in this way almost as soon as spray cans appeared. Users have tried almost every type of aerosol product—insecticides, disinfectants, hair sprays, furniture polish, even non-stick pan coaters.

The main categories of inhalants that are abused and their active ingredients are:

Inhalant	Active Ingredient
Glues and paint thinners	toluene, hexane, acetone, methyl alcohol, trichloroethylene, ethyl acetate
Lighter fluid	naptha
Aerosols	fluorinated hydrocarbons, nitrous oxide
Cleaning solutions	trichloroethylene, carbon tetrachloride
Gasoline	benzene
Amyl nitrate	amyl nitrate
Butyl Nitrate	butyl nitrate
Nitrous oxide	nitrous oxide

VOLATILE SOLVENTS AND AEROSOLS

METHOD OF ACTION

The inhaled vapors pass through the lungs into the bloodstream, and on to the brain, where they quickly cross the blood brain barrier. The immediate short-term effect is a mild intoxication similar to alcohol, followed by brief euphoria lasting from a few minutes to an hour, with excitement and delusions of strength and power. The user may lose consciousness during or after this period.

METHOD OF ABUSE

The most common method of use is direct sniffing. Some users enhance the effect by increasing the concentration of the vapor. A quantity of the substance is put into a plastic or paper bag, which is placed over the face. The fumes are then breathed in until intoxication is achieved. Alternatively, a plastic bag is placed over the head and the substance sniffed directly from the container. A trashcan liner may also be used, and then the entire head and shoulders are covered. Solvents may also be poured onto cloths and sniffed, and aerosols are either sprayed into containers or inhaled straight from the can.

BEHAVIORAL AND PSYCHOLOGICAL EFFECTS

During the "high," the user experiences intoxication, euphoria, excitement, delusions of strength and power, visual distortions, loss of coordination and judgment, slurred speech, and giddiness. Hallucinations may occur with high doses. Because the effects are disinhibiting, aggressiveness and violent behavior are not uncommon if the user doesn't fall asleep first. There may be uncontrolled giggling, a vacant stare, mental confusion, and antisocial behavior. Eventually, school performance and social life suffer dramatically.

Occasionally users will continue to sniff until they are seriously intoxicated, making them unaware of everyday hazards and putting them at risk for accidents. Finally they may become drowsy or unconscious, in which case falling, or choking on their own vomit, can lead to sudden death.

PHYSICAL EFFECTS

Regular users suffer from headaches, drowsiness, and irritability. Long-term or chronic use may lead to "sniffer's rash" around the nose and mouth, conjunctivitis, liver and kidney damage, cardiac irregularities, and in extreme cases damage to the brain and peripheral nervous system. There may be a chemical smell on the breath.

A number of studies have shown impaired memory, movement-coordination problems, impaired language skills, poor ability to process information, and a diminished ability to think abstractly in chronic inhalant abusers. These are all signs of possible permanent brain damage. Abuse can also cause the destruction of bone marrow, digestive disorders, anemia, convulsions, and certain types of leukemia.

EFFECTS ON PREGNANCY

The use of solvents during pregnancy has been linked to central nervous system defects in newborns. Mental retardation and abnormal facial features also have been seen in babies whose mothers used inhalants or solvents in combination with alcohol while they were pregnant. Chemicals can show up in the milk of lactating users.

DOSAGES

No source has reliable figures on the doses used in inhalant abuse, because users take in arbitrary amounts, and chemical strengths differ from product to product.

TOXIC EFFECTS AND OVERDOSE

In addition to brain, liver, kidney, and bone marrow damage, individual solvents are known to have specific toxic effects:

- **Methyl alcohol:** Headaches, weakness, delayed blindness (up to 30 hours after use), death.

- **Hexane:** Anemia, nerve degeneration, muscle weakness, patches of numbness.

- **Trichloroethylene:** Liver damage, kidney damage, damage to optic and other cranial nerves, death.

- **Toluene:** Nausea, stomach pain, loss of appetite, jaundice, enlarged liver, urinary dysfunction, kidney damage, mental dullness, tremors, emotional disturbances, staggering, nerve and brain damage.

- **Ethyl acetate:** Severe eye, skin and mucous membrane irritation, severe depression of the central nervous system.

- **Ketones:** Same as ethyl acetate but the substance is also highly flammable.

The inherent dangers of inhalant use include accidents from falls, car accidents, industrial accidents, accidental death by suffocation (if user loses consciousness while the plastic bag is over his head), choking on vomit, spraying aerosol containers or gases directly into the nose or mouth (causing asphyxiation), and cardiac arrest. The further danger of burns and explosions comes when the substance is heated over a fire or other naked heat source.

TOLERANCE, ADDICTION, AND WITHDRAWAL

There is no evidence of significant physical dependence, but chronic users who abruptly stop abusing these agents sometimes experience: stomach pain; headache; a numbness and tingling in the hands, feet, and other parts of the body; disorientation; memory impairment; problems with coordination; hallucinations; delusions; feelings of persecution; and slurred speech.

Strong psychological dependence on these drugs develops quickly, and chronic users find it hard to stop. Tolerance to a particular solvent occurs rapidly, although this does not cause a cross-tolerance to other types of solvents. When people do stop abusing solvents without proper treatment, they often start abusing other drugs such as alcohol and depressants.

OPTIONS FOR TREATMENT

Users should first be checked by a medical doctor to determine the extent of physical and psychological damage. It is often difficult to get inhalant abusers into a treatment program due to the combined effects of low socioeconomic status, family problems, school failures, antisocial behavior, and brain damage. If family or friends can get help, a therapeutic community or outpatient program featuring counseling and drug education are advised. Behavior modification techniques are helpful for chronic users.

Because inhalant abusers often have strong feelings of inferiority and deep-rooted emotional problems, many experts advise long-term psychotherapy once the addiction has been treated in order to prevent relapses of destructive behavior. (See Chapter Twenty-Four for more information about drug treatment programs.)

LONG-TERM PROGNOSIS

Physically, much of the damage to body and mind suffered by a chronic abuser of these agents can be permanent. The prognosis for staying off these drugs, or drugs in general, depends on the life situation of the patient. If the person has strong personal resources and receives good treatment, he or she may not go on to abuse other drugs. But if the person comes from a poor socioeconomic background, with no support from family or friends, the outlook is bleak. In these cases, inhalant abuse will either continue or may be followed by other types of chemical dependency.

AMYL AND BUTYL NITRATE

METHOD OF ACTION

Amyl nitrate was used before 1960 to relieve the symptoms of angina pectoris because of its action as a vasodilator (a chemical that expands blood vessels). It was taken off the controlled prescription drug list of the Food and Drug Administration when more sophisticated medications came into use. It was reinstated in the listings in 1969, when word came of its abuse by adolescents, who were obtaining it illegally. However, at that point its non-prescription chemical cousins, butyl nitrate and isobutyl nitrate, became widely available, eventually as legal room deodorizers sold in "head shops" (stores selling drug paraphernalia) with the names "Locker Room" and "Rush." These drugs first gained popularity because of their reputation for enhancing sex.

METHOD OF ABUSE
Plastic bags are sometimes used to inhale these substances, which come in small bottles, but some users carry their own sniffing devices.

BEHAVIORAL AND PSYCHOLOGICAL EFFECTS
Effects are felt in under 30 seconds and last for about 3 minutes. Users feel lightheaded and giddy, with some distortion of perception. Time seems to stretch and sensory stimulation appears more intense (hence, its use just before sexual orgasm). Since these drugs do have disinhibiting effects, the person may exhibit aggressive behavior.

PHYSICAL EFFECTS
Nausea, dizziness, flushing, and occasional loss of consciousness have been experienced.

EFFECTS ON PREGNANCY
Pregnant and lactating women are advised against the use of any inhalant, which has been linked to birth defects.

DOSAGES
See *VOLATILE SOLVENTS AND AEROSOLS*, pages 207-210.

TOXIC EFFECTS AND OVERDOSE
More toxic effects include vomiting, a weakened pulse rate, and loss of coordination. The expansion of blood vessels serving the brain can cause severe headaches and even stroke-like incidents. When used with alcohol, the chance of adverse effects increases dramatically. These drugs are very dangerous for people with low blood pressure, recent head injuries, or glaucoma (because of increased pressure in the eye). Death from overdose is not common, but in susceptible people it is possible.

TOLERANCE, ADDICTION, AND WITHDRAWAL
As with any inhalant, tolerance builds up, and the user can become psychologically addicted.

OPTIONS FOR TREATMENT
People who abuse these inhalants often use other drugs, such as alcohol,

hallucinogens, or depressants. An inpatient treatment program is advised in such cases, with drug education and counseling.

LONG-TERM PROGNOSIS

Susceptible people can sustain permanent physical (in the case of stroke-like incidents) and mental damage from the abuse of these drugs. Adolescents who go through a "phase" and use this drug alone usually recover without problems. People who have multiple dependencies are more difficult to treat, unless they have strong personal resources.

NITROUS OXIDE

METHOD OF ACTION

Although classed with inhalants, nitrous oxide is a mild anesthetic with strong analgesic (pain-killing) properties. Some people are acquainted with it by the term "laughing gas." It is still used in medicine—principally dentistry. It also is a propellant for aerosol whipped cream. It goes to work within seconds of being inhaled, and the "high" can last for 3 or more minutes. A sense of well-being may remain for several hours.

METHOD OF ABUSE

Nitrous oxide is sold in small metal cylinders called "whippets," along with the balloon needed for inhalation. Users fill up the balloon with nitrous oxide and inhale it from the balloon. If a regular tank is being used, an anesthetic mask is held or strapped onto the head.

BEHAVIORAL AND PSYCHOLOGICAL EFFECTS

Users feel exhilirated, and sometimes laugh uncontrollably. They may lose consciousness for a few seconds, and before going under experience the feeling of flying. Sensory distortion is possible once consciousness returns.

PHYSICAL EFFECTS

Mild nausea and a dry throat are the only physical side effects.

EFFECTS ON PREGNANCY

While pregnant women and nursing mothers are not advised to abuse this—or any other—drug, there is little information at the present time concerning the effects of nitrous oxide on pregnancy and lactation.

DOSAGES
See *VOLATILE SOLVENTS AND AEROSOLS*, pages 207-210.

TOXIC EFFECTS AND OVERDOSE
Nitrous oxide is non-toxic, but it is dangerous. Users have died, mainly through accidents. A frostbite reaction occurs when a person tries to draw the gas directly from the cylinder, causing frozen noses, lips, mouths, throats, and vocal cords. People can suffer serious fractures if they lose consciousness while standing, and anyone driving or operating machinery under the influence of the drug is at great risk.

Strapping on an anesthetic mask to take the drug can have more serious consequences. Nitrous oxide does not provide all the oxygen the brain needs (anesthesiologists mix it with 30 percent pure oxygen), so some users who have lost consciousness under the mask have either suffocated or suffered brain damage.

TOLERANCE, ADDICTION, AND WITHDRAWAL
It is not common today, as it was in the 19th century, for people to chronically abuse nitrous oxide. But an increasing tolerance and psychological addiction are possible for those who make this their drug of choice.

OPTIONS FOR TREATMENT
People who abuse nitrous oxide must be treated like any chronic user of inhalants. (Abusers may be health professionals, who have easier access to the drug, tank and mask.) A comprehensive inpatient program is advised, and if the problem becomes serious, hospitalization may also be needed.

LONG-TERM PROGNOSIS
If permanent brain damage has not been sustained, personal resources are good, other drugs are not abused as well, and if the person receives proper treatment, there is every reason for optimism.

CHAPTER TWENTY-FOUR

Options for Treatment

Drug dependency is not incurable, as it was once thought to be. In fact, with the proper programs and strong personal motivation, more than 75 percent of previously addicted people recover completely and go on to lead normal, productive lives. This is mainly because more types of treatment exist today than ever before, and more doctors and counselors are experienced in coping with the problems of drug abuse.

Although we have discussed treatments for specific drug dependencies in preceding chapters, it is worthwhile to discuss them again in greater detail. Our goal is to give drug abusers and/or their families and friends a clear picture of how their problems might be solved.

Dependency is the same no matter what the socioeconomic class, so the process of getting off and staying off drugs is also essentially the same. It is true that strong personal resources—a fulfilling job, a good education, a comfortable home, and strong family ties—can help a great deal, but all people who truly want to become drug-free can be helped toward achieving that goal.

The first step any dependent person must make is the admission that he or she has a drug problem. Denial is characteristic of drug abusers.

"I can handle it."

"I can stop anytime I want to."

"I'm not that stupid."

These statements are frequently made by seriously dependent people. They may be saying these things to get friends and family members to leave them alone, or they may honestly believe them, unable to admit the truth—even to themselves. Often, they believe they need the drug to function normally, and are desperately afraid of existing without it. In other cases, the pains of withdrawal are truly frightening, and the reinforcement that comes from taking more of the drug eases the aches and fears.

When the drug user or his family finally decides to seek help, the first step should be to see a doctor—often the family doctor. A physician can determine if the drug has seriously harmed body or mind. The doctor can also find out if the drug abuse has been used to mask a physical or emotional illness. Some people start taking drugs because of conditions such as chronic back pain, and chemically depressed people may turn to cocaine or other stimulants to relieve the constant "blues."

Chronic drug abusers are often malnourished, and may be suffering from serious vitamin and/or mineral deficiencies. The family doctor can determine if this is the case and prescribe appropriate nutritional therapy. Finally, the family doctor is often the best source for the name of a good drug treatment program.

DETOXIFICATION

Drugs with the highest potential for addiction are opioids, depressants, and stimulants (particularly cocaine). People trying to withdraw from these drugs often need close medical supervision. If drug involvement has been serious, the first step is usually detoxification.

Detoxification is the process of gradually withdrawing a drug from someone who is physically or psychologically dependent on it, either by administering decreasing amounts of the drug or by substituting another drug with the same effects. This type of program may be necessary as a first step, but addicted people and their families must remember that detoxification alone is too limited to cure the user. He must have in-depth, ongoing counseling and support to remain permanently drug-free.

"Detox" programs start by determining the user's level of tolerance (and identifying any illnesses, injuries, and physical or emotional conditions) in order to establish the dosage needed to prevent withdrawal symptoms. This is particularly crucial in depressant withdrawal, which can be life-threatening, but all types of severe withdrawal are best avoided if possible. Users who suffer debilitating withdrawal symptoms are more prone to relapse. After all, the quickest and easiest way to stop the pain is to resume taking the drug. For these reasons, going "cold turkey" (abruptly stopping use of the drug) is not favored by many experts when dealing with opioid or depressant abuse.

Doctors use either methadone (a synthetic narcotic) or a non-narcotic psychoactive to detoxify heroin or morphine addicts. Usually, a 10 percent reduction in dosage over a certain period of time (a day, a week) is employed until total abstinence is achieved.

For multiple drug abusers, the detoxification process is more complex. People dependent on narcotics and sedatives are usually withdrawn from the sedatives first, while receiving enough methadone to prevent withdrawal symptoms. The use of methadone, a highly addictive opioid narcotic, is controversial in itself. Many doctors feel that it should be used as a last resort, only when other forms of treatment have failed, since it is also a potential drug of abuse. Today, the antihypertensive drug clonidine (Catapres) offers new hope for the opiate addict, in that it is the first non-addictive, non-narcotic treatment for opiate withdrawal. It fools the brain into thinking it's not in withdrawal when it is. Using this drug, a person addicted to heroin or methadone may be drug-free in 10-14 days.

For cocaine users, detox is usually done without chemical support, although some patients may be given antidepressants or lithium if their depression or manic-depression is endogenous (of physiological origin) and it predates their use of cocaine. Certain drugs such as bromocriptine help reduce cravings and drug urges among cocaine users. This drug, which is usually employed in the treatment of Parkinson's disease, seems to mask the withdrawal symptoms caused by depletion of the neurotransmitter dopamine.

Because withdrawal from sedatives and hypnotics is often severe and life-threatening, it rarely should be attempted outside a hospital.

Users and/or their families should look for an established detoxification unit with an experienced team in a teaching hospital, or similar institution. If your family doctor cannot recommend one, there is a list of numbers to call at the end of this chapter, many of which can help you locate treatment centers of all kinds in your area.

One note of caution, however: It is best to stay away from most quasi-religious or politically oriented programs. Their procedures may come dangerously close to "brainwashing," and their staffs may be trying to substitute one type of addiction for another. Their ultimate goal may be to convert the already weakened drug user to their ideologies. This is not the type of pressure and confusion a recovering drug abuser needs.

RESIDENTIAL PROGRAMS AND OUTPATIENT TREATMENT

After detoxification, or if it is not needed, a choice for long-term treatment must be made. These are the types of programs designed to keep the user off drugs on a permanent basis. Staying off drugs is a lifelong process.

Basically, there are two major types of treatment—residential and outpatient. If the user has strong personal resources and productive employment, an outpatient program is usually best. But for those without jobs, families, or who are suffering from profound drug involvement, a residential program may be more successful.

One of the most popular forms of resident treatment is a *therapeutic community (TC)*, such as the programs run by Phoenix House in New York and California. TC's work like large families providing mutual support. Every resident has a job of some sort—working in the kitchen, cleaning, painting, or doing repairs. Some of the TC's staff members are former drug abusers trained in clinical methods. They serve as proof to the others that the program works. Psychological counseling focuses more on life-changing strategies and current problems than it does on delving into childhood incidents to find the cause of problems. The longer a drug abuser remains in the TC, the better the chances for a cure and an improvement of psychological problems.

If you are considering a TC, make sure it is licensed or approved by the state's drug abuse agency, and that it is voluntary and not based on physical coercion. For a referral, you or your doctor can contact a drug abuse service or state agency that handles treatment services. For example, the state of California has a division called the Department of Alcohol and Drug Programs.

Outpatient, drug-free programs (OPDF) can range from drop-in "rap" centers to free clinics to highly structured programs. The ones that emphasize group therapy, individual counseling, drug education, and which involve family members are best for people with jobs, responsibilities, and less serious drug dependencies. At the start of these programs, urine and blood may be tested several times a week, so a climate of trust can be established between user and counselor. There is often a contractual agreement, which stipulates that if the person doesn't stay off drugs, he will be hospitalized. Many programs use a three-phase system:

Phase I, or the phase of initial abstinence, can last 30-90 days or more. During this time, patients are seen by a counselor every day for support and education.

Phase II, or relapse prevention, involves lifestyle-changing strategies. Ex-users are encouraged to break off associations with friends and peers who are drug users, to find new activities and interests to fill their time, to get their bodies and minds in shape through exercise and relaxation techniques, and to set new, productive goals for their lives.

Phase III, or consolidation, usually starts after the first year, and involves participation in group therapy or a self-help group such as Cocaine Anonymous or Pills Anonymous. These are modeled after Alcoholics Anonymous and supervised by qualified people. Some ex-users choose to stay in such a group for many years.

OTHER TYPES OF TREATMENT

In recent years, the Chinese method of *acupuncture* has given considerable relief to some people dependent on cocaine or narcotics, and may be useful for all types of drug addiction. Its ability to control withdrawal may be due to some unknown neurochemical activity and the possibility that it stimulates the production of natural endorphins—the brain-made chemicals often called the body's "morphine."

Antagonist therapy, which has not been very successful, is used to treat narcotics abusers. It is the use of one drug to block the effects of another by antagonist action. For instance, if the patient takes heroin and gets no reinforcement (pleasure), then the reason for taking the drug vanishes. Antagonists work in the brain by moving in on receptor sites so that the drug of abuse cannot make a connection. Users trying this type of program must first be detoxified.

Although cyclazocine, the first narcotic antagonist used, blocks heroin for about 24 hours, its side effects are weakness, fatigue, tension, and possible mental confusion. Naloxone has none of these effects but is too short-acting to be of use. Naltrexone is now being tried; it can be taken orally and blocks heroin for 24 hours.

Behavior modification is the attempt to change patterns of behavior that lead to drug use, and employs techniques such as relaxation exercises and hypnosis. Desirable behavior may also be "bought" with rewards appropriate to the setting. For example, prisoner-addicts are sometimes offered an earlier release date if they attend group therapy and drug education programs.

"Counterconditioning" employs a drug that causes vomiting, such as apomorphine or ipecac, which is given to a user with his drug of dependence to recondition him. His association with drug use becomes one of suffering and nausea, rather than pleasure. Hypnosis may also be used to link drug use with nausea, anxiety, and unpleasant feelings.

Contingency contracting, which was mentioned in Chapter Fifteen, is a new form of treatment that has shown tremendous success with cocaine abusers in the few places it has been used. Here, the user literally blackmails himself. At the start of treatment, he writes several letters, to employers, friends, licensing boards—any place that could cause him emotional or financial harm. These letters admit to drug abuse. He may also write checks (contributions) to causes he despises. These letters or checks are then put in the hands of the program supervisors, and the patient is told they will be mailed out if he doesn't stay clear of drugs for a set period of time (usually 3 months).

Electrotherapy was developed by Scottish surgeon Margaret Patterson. It is often called NeuroElectric Therapy (NET) and is used for rapid detoxification from narcotics abuse. A box-like device, which clips onto the user's belt, sends an electric current through wires to tiny electrodes placed over the mastoid bones behind the ears. The technique resembles, and is based on, the use of acupuncture with electrical stimulation. The electricity is at very low levels and the whole procedure, which is still controversial, works best when combined with counseling and a stable environment.

STAYING OFF

While the physical symptoms of withdrawal may be gone in a few days to a few weeks, the psychological pains may be longer-lasting. Ex-users often feel depressed, angry, anxious, bored, restless, and empty for a long period of time. Their physical health and nutritional status may have been compromised during the period of drug abuse. These problems must be dealt with if a person is to lead a completely drug-free life. Formerly dependent people must come to understand how harmful drug abuse is, and stay away from people and situations that lead to drug taking.

All ex-users should take a simple one-per-day multiple vitamin preparation (megadoses are not advised and can be dangerous) and eat balanced meals. Exercise is vital to recondition and relax the body. Weight-lifting and swimming are good ways to relieve tension. Long-distance running often works well for ex-cocaine users: the runner's "high" that results resembles the feeling produced by the drug.

Learning new relaxation techniques, such as stretching exercises, simple meditation, yoga, and biofeedback, are very useful. Finding new hobbies, such as cooking or photography, can take a person's mind off drugs. Education or new employment is another way. Ex-users should try to fill up their time with appointments, jobs, and assignments, because idle hours can lead to drug cravings and depression.

However, the recovering drug abuser and his or her family must realize that these changes cannot be made overnight. It may be a slow process of rebuilding one's life, requiring several years and a healthy dose of support and guidance from friends, family, and professional counselors.

Family and loved ones can help immensely through encouragement, or even through confrontation if they suspect that drug abuse has resumed. When drug use is tolerated, it is not a sign of love; it is complicity.

In choosing a drug-treatment program, families should visit with staff members, check references, investigate the program's history, and ask financial questions about insurance coverage, the length of stay that will be covered, and any hidden costs. They must also understand that long-term hospitalization or residential treatment may be the only way to keep loved ones permanently drug-free, especially in cases of compulsive drug use, physiological dependency that presents psychiatric and physical problems, severe impairment of social functioning, strong resistance to treatment, or failure in outpatient programs,.

Programs have different levels of success, and some drugs are easier to "kick" than others. But in the long run, it is the individual's motivation to get off and stay off drugs that makes the difference.

WHERE TO CALL FOR HELP

National Clearinghouse for Drug Abuse Information (NCDAI)
301-443-6500

Phoenix House Foundation
212-595-5810

The American Council for Drug Education (ACDE)
301-984-5700
212-758-8060

Pyramid   800-638-2045

National Institute on Drug Abuse (NIDA)
U.S. Department of Health and Human Services
800-638-2045
301-443-1124

NIDA Hotline
800-662-HELP

Cocaine Hotline
800-COCAINE

Division of Substance Abuse Services
800-522-5353

Drug Enforcement Administration (DEA)
Washington Field Division
202-724-7834

Do It Now Foundation
602-257-0797

State Agencies, such as:
Department of Alcohol and Drug Abuse
Department of Health Services
Department of Human Services
Department of Mental Health
Substance Abuse Services

Listings for:
Alcoholics Anonymous
Narcotics Anonymous
Cocaine Anonymous
Pills Anonymous
Local affiliates of the National Council on Alcoholism
Local health departments
Community hospitals, free clinics
Social service agencies

Bibliography

BOOKS

Barnhart, Edward R. *Physician's Desk Reference*, 39th ed. New Jersey: Medical Economics Company, 1985.

Bassuk, E. L., Schoonover, S. C., and Gelenberg, A. J., eds. *The Practitioner's Guide to Psychoactive Drugs*, 2nd ed. New York and London: Plenum Medical Book Company, 1983.

Berne, Eric. *A Layman's Guide to Psychiatry and Psychoanalysis*. New York: Ballantine Books, 1957.

British Dental Assoc., British Medical Assoc., and The Pharmaceutical Society of Great Britain. *Dental Practitioners' Formulary together with British National Formulary*. London: The British Medical Assoc. and the Pharmaceutical Society of Great Britain, 1984.

Chatlos, Calvin. *Crack: What You Should Know About the Cocaine Epidemic*. New York: Perigee Books, The Putman Publishing Group, 1987.

Chilnick, Lawrence, ed. *The Little Black Pill Book*. New York: Bantam Books, 1983.

Chilnick, Lawrence, et. al., eds. *The Coke Book*. New York: Berkley Books, 1984.

Coleman, J. C., Butcher J. N., and Carson, R. C. *Abnormal Psychology and Modern Life*, 7th ed. Illinois, Texas, New Jersey, California, Georgia and London, England: Scott, Foresman and Company, 1984.

DuPont, R. L. Jr. *Getting Tough on Gateway Drugs*. Washington, D.C.: American Psychiatric Press, Inc., 1984.

Duquesne, T. and Reeves, J. *A Handbook of Psychoactive Medicines*. London: Quartet Books, 1982.

Fieve, Ronald R. *Moodswing*. New York: Bantam Books, 1975.

Gilman, Alfred G. and Goodman, Louis S., eds. *The Pharmacological Basis of Therapeutics*, 7th ed. New York: Macmillan Publishing Company, 1985.

Good, W. V., and Nelson, J. E. *Psychiatry Made Ridiculously Simple*. Miami: Medmaster, 1984.

Hoover, R. D., ed. *Drugs of Abuse*. U. S. Government Printing Office, DEA, 1985.

Julien, Robert M. *A Primer of Drug Action*, 4th ed. New York: W. H. Freeman and Company, 1985.

Kaplan, Harold I. and Sadock, Benjamin J. *Modern Synopsis of Comprehensive Textbook of Psychiatry/IV*. Baltimore: Williams & Wilkins, 1985.

Klein, Donald F., Gittelman, Rachel, Quitkin, Frederic, and Rifkin, Arthur. *Diagnosis and Drug Treatment of Psychiatric Disorders: Adults and Children*, 2nd ed. Baltimore: Williams & Wilkins, 1980.

Maxmen, Jerrold S. *The New Psychiatry*. New York: William Morrow and Company, 1985.

Morgan, Brian L. G. *The Food & Drug Interaction Guide*. New York: Simon and Schuster, 1986.

Morgan, Brian L. G. and Morgan, Roberta. *Brainfood*. Tucson, Arizona: The Body Press/HPBooks, 1987.

Mothner, I. and Weitz, A. *How to Get Off Drugs*. New York: Rolling Stone Press/Simon and Schuster, 1984.

Rowe, Clarence J. *An Outline of Psychiatry*. Iowa: Wm. C. Brown Publishers, 1984.

Spitzer, Robert L., Skodol, Andrew E., Gibbon, Miriam, and Williams, Janet B. W. *DSM-III Case Book.* Washington, D.C.: American Psychiatric Association, 1981.

Stockley, D. *Drug Warning.* London and Sydney: Macdonald & Co., Ltd., 1986.

Waldinger, Robert J. *Psychiatry for Medical Students.* Washington, D.C.: American Psychiatric Press, 1984.

Washton, A. M. *Crack: What You Need To Know.* Florida: Health Communications, Inc., 1986.

Wolman, Benjamin B., ed. *The Therapist's Handbook.* New York: Van Nostrand Reinhold, 1976.

ARTICLES AND PAMPHLETS
Pamphlets from the American Council for Drug Education (ACDE):
   "Drugs and Pregnancy"
   "Treating Marijuana Dependency"
   "The Therapeutic Potentials of Marijuana's Components"
   "Marijuana"
   "Marijuana and the Lungs"
   "Treating the Marijuana-Dependent Person"
   "Cocaine Treatment: A Guide"
   "Cocaine: Some Questions and Answers"
   "Crack: Some Questions and Answers"

"Cocaine Use in America," *Prevention Networks*, National Institute on Drug Abuse, U. S. Government Printing Office, April 1986, pp. 1-16.

"Controlled Substances Analogs," Drug Control Section, Drug Enforcement Administration (DEA), 1986.

"Crack," *TIME Magazine*, June 2, 1986, pp. 16-18.

"Designer Drugs," *Science 85*, March, pp. 61-67.

"Designer Drugs," *Street Pharmacologist*, Vol. VIII, Nos. 5-6, May-June 1985, Up Front, Inc.

Pamphlets from Do It Now (D.I.N.) Publications, Phoenix, Arizona:
   "MDA/MDM: The Chemical Pursuit of Ecstasy," 1985.
   "Designer Drugs," 1984.
   "Crystal, Crank, & Speedy Stuff," 1981.

"Drugs: The Enemy Within," *TIME Magazine*, Sept. 15, 1986, pp. 60-68.

"MDMA: Psychedelic Drug Faces Regulation," *Psychology Today*, May 1985, pp. 68-69.

"Report on Crack," New York State, Division of Substance Abuse Services, 1986.

"Special Report: The Crack Situation in the United States," Drug Enforcement Administration (DEA), Washington, D.C., 1986.

"The Health Implications of Marijuana Use," U. S. Department of Justice, DEA, July 1985.

"The New Drug They Call 'Ecstasy,'" *New York Magazine*, May 20, 1985, pp. 38-43.

Index